Understanding Asperger Syndrome and High Functioning Autism

Autism Spectrum Disorders Library

Series Editor: Gary B. Mesibov

UNDERSTANDING ASPERGER SYNDROME AND HIGH
FUNCTIONING AUTISM
Gary B. Mesibov, Victoria Shea, and Lynn W. Adams

A Continuation Order Plan is available for this series. A continuation order will bring delivery
of each new volume immediately upon publication. Volumes are billed only upon actual
shipment. For further information please contact the publisher.

Understanding Asperger Syndrome and High Functioning Autism

Gary B. Mesibov and
Victoria Shea
University of North Carolina
Chapel Hill, North Carolina

and

Lynn W. Adams
Mercy Family Center
New Orleans, Louisiana

Kluwer Academic / Plenum Publishers
New York, Boston, Dordrecht, London, Moscow

ISBN 0-306-46626-0 (Hardbound)
ISBN 0-306-46627-9 (Paperback)

© 2001 Kluwer Academic/Plenum Publishers, New York
233 Spring Street, New York, New York 10013

http://www.wkap.nl/

10 9 8 7 6 5 4 3 2 1

A C.I.P. record for this book is available from the Library of Congress

Printed in the United States of America

Preface

This volume is designed to provide an overview of Asperger's Syndrome/High Functioning Autism for professionals, parents, and others concerned about these conditions. It is part of the library series that has been created for the many people interested in the field of autism spectrum disorders who want up-to-date, authoritative information without having to locate and read through the original sources. Our goal in this series is to review, synthesize, and organize the information so that it can be presented comprehensively and clearly.

This volume is the culmination of over a decade of clinical work identifying, organizing, writing, and editing the most current information available about this high functioning group of people with autism spectrum disorders from current reputable sources. The book explores the history and emphasizes the diagnosis, assessment, and treatment of these people and their families. We hope that we have done justice to this extensive literature so that it can be of use to these people themselves as well as to their many friends, colleagues, and families, and to the interested citizens who are seeking more information about this intriguing area of inquiry.

Acknowledgments

We are indebted to many people for their help on this project, and we want to acknowledge their substantial contributions. First and foremost we want to thank our TEACCH colleagues and the many families and professionals who have worked with us. Their interest in our views, perceptive comments about HFA/AS, their support, and their assistance have been invaluable. There are many exciting and rewarding aspects of living and working in North Carolina, but most important are the terrific people we meet and work with.

Joan Berry has been particularly important throughout this project, typing numerous drafts, changes, corrections, and insertions. She has done all of this work with a smile on her face and her usual accuracy and efficiency. Leia Grossman, a student research assistant, did many of the mundane tasks that are so essential for an accurate and comprehensive final product. Her assistance in tracking down and checking references has added immeasurably to this final product.

Finally, as with all our projects collaborating with Kluwer, our editor, Mariclaire Cloutier, has to be thanked for her responsiveness, assistance, and all-around excellence. Her patience as we wrote and rewrote the final drafts is especially appreciated.

Finally, our friends, families, and colleagues are to be thanked for enduring our absence as we worked the demanding schedule that a project like this requires. Their interest and understanding made all of this bearable, even during the most intense periods of working on this manuscript. Special thanks are due to Joan Goodrich Lang for her ongoing interest and support.

Contents

Asperger Syndrome/ High Functioning Autism

Reflections by a 52-year-old prodigious savant on being one, and prospects for future research on his peers. I write this on the 2732nd Thursday of my life. I was born exactly two years after Bill Clinton, but I inhaled Asperger's Syndrome. Since the end of first grade, when I became a local town curiosity, I have exhibited several skills that stood in stark contrast to my general awkwardness, social clumsiness, and hypersensitive posture.

My first noticed skill was an ability to parrot back songs immediately after my music teacher sang them. Once I knew how to read music, I instantly saw the music, for each instrument, roll by, mentally, for most music that I heard. I could play melodies back, one-handed, on a piano, but two hands was a disaster and besides, my family did not have a piano so that was out.

However, extreme stage fright discouraged me from much use of this talent and it became a private way to nod out of class. It was more fun, since I read about four times as fast as my peers, to kill time listening to classical music, than it was to gain unpopularity by impatiently leering at my classmates, tapping my fingers until they finished their reading chores.

The next noticeable skill was numbers. My father discovered what I could do and showed me off to my Mom, a substitute eighth grade math teacher. I was next, being shown off, in school, to every new student, with the command, "just give him any two numbers and watch what happens." Considering that most of my peers were impressed by three or four digit numbers, that was not hard to satisfy. I was able then and still am able to do multiplication, division, roots of all sizes and eventually other functions, change number bases, etc., as soon as I knew what these operations were.

The problem with this was that people thought I was good at math. This is not math. This is just calculating. Math is a lot more abstract and my eventual problem with abstractions got to me in late college, when I began to take graduate level math classes. The moral of that is that, while it is nice to see a special skill appear, it is necessary to know what it is and what it isn't.

My last special skill, shared by the rest of my male family peers, is an excellent memory, long-term and very visual. My father never needed a map to go anywhere he had been, no matter how long ago. He often remembered the layouts of buildings after one visit. My oldest brother won his first academic prize for an Astronomy project and my middle brother has been an art director in the movie industry for thirty years. As for me, many people have always marveled at my memory.

In college, it got me in "trouble." I was in a very small, unorthodox fraternity. It was rush week, when we looked for new members. The University of Michigan had a "Freshman Directory." This had most of the new class, each with a photo, brief bio, hometown, major, hobbies, etc. I casually looked at it one night before rush week began.

The next afternoon, it was about 1:20 and a young man appeared at my house's front door. He was late and I opened up the door and helped him with his coat. Two brothers wanted to get him going on a house tour and didn't wait for him to get a name tag. I looked at his face and saw it just as it appeared in the Freshman directory.

As my brothers led him upstairs, I shouted, "Fred, you need a name tag!" and rushed up to give a proper tag with his full name, campus address, hometown, and major. He looked at me and asked, "How do you know all of this about me?" I knew I was caught, and just blushed, saying, "It was all in the directory." My two brothers smiled, looked at Fred and me and said, "We'll have to explain Brother Newport to you, later."

Fred finished his house tour, got his coat, and never came back. He pledged a house down the block and periodically, I saw him enrolled there, with his new pledge brothers, and would shout, "Fred!" from across the street. Once, he kind of waved back, probably wondering if I worked for the FBI.

So, that is why I am a prodigious talented savant. It has been a mixed blessing. Like most savants, I struggled most of my life in the most menial of jobs and living arrangements and had little in the way of relationships. Only with mentors, proper diet, and exercise have I had any real improvement. – Jerry Newport, 12/00

INTRODUCTION

First identified in the professional literature by Leo Kanner and Hans Asperger in 1943 and 1944, autism/Asperger Syndrome (AS) remained primarily of interest to professionals working with these children and their families for the next four decades. This changed in 1988 with the release of the film *Rain Man*. Dustin Hoffman's remarkable portrayal of Raymond, a capable young man with autism, captured the interest of viewers all over the world. Because of this film, the general public's knowledge of, and interest in, autism increased, as did the demand for more information about autism/AS.

Some of the reasons why *Rain Man* generated so much public interest are similar to reasons professionals are so frequently fascinated by this disability or why we find Jerry Newport's opening paragraph so intriguing. First, there are the remarkable contrasts between areas of near normal functioning and severe disabilities. Although Raymond had a peculiar gait and an unusual way of pronouncing words, he could talk, interact, care for most of his daily needs, and function in the community. On the other hand, his relationships were unusual and his coping strategies quite limited. Filmgoers were impressed by the contrasts between his positive and tender relationship with his brother and his unusual interactions with the women he met in Las Vegas. Other telling contrasts were between his generally appropriate behaviors in many community settings and his tantrum at the airport and his panic at the prospect of missing his favorite television show. How can someone be so similar to the rest of us in his behavior and level of functioning in some situations, yet so different in many others?

Rain Man's extraordinary skills have also piqued many curiosities. An uneven profile of strengths and weaknesses is a common characteristic of autism/AS, and, at times, the strengths can be remarkable. Some of the most compelling scenes in the film revolve around Raymond's extraordinary abilities. We marvel at Raymond's memory when he is able to recall numbers from the telephone book he browses through in his hotel room. Raymond's multiplying 3-digit numbers in his head faster than the psychiatrist can compute them with his calculator is another memorable image. This scene actually helped another young man with autism to seek his own diagnosis in his mid-30s. Watching this scene, Jerry Newport told Leslie Stahl on a TV interview on *60 Minutes*, encouraged him to pursue a diagnostic evaluation because he was able to compute the figures more rapidly than Raymond was able to generate the answers on the screen. Raymond's special skills are also featured during the scene in the restaurant when he is able to count in a matter of milliseconds the number of toothpicks in a pile that fall from his table.

Raymond is also interesting to many of us because of his idiosyncratic behaviors. Perhaps these are so interesting because they are so unusual, but equally likely they remind us of our own idiosyncracies, exaggerated to an extreme that is comical and endearing. For example, Raymond's obsessive concern with his favorite TV show or his need to buy a certain brand of underwear at K-Mart are scenes that millions of viewers enjoyed and can still easily relate to their own experiences.

Raymond is a person with a particular form of autism that is associated with many well-developed skills. Some professionals would label this "Asperger Syndrome" (AS), while others might use the term "high functioning autism" (HFA). The term "high functioning autism" is not technically a diagnosis in any official diagnostic system. Rather, it is used informally and descriptively for autism not associated with mental retardation (that is, IQ of 70 or above). Some professionals use AS and HFA interchangeably, while others argue that these are different, although related, conditions.

This book will explore what is known about AS/HFA and explain current theories and practice. Starting with an historical summary of the early recognition and formulations of the disorder, the book will then explore diagnostic issues, psychological assessment, current treatment practices, and other substantive issues. We intend to maintain the fascination and wonder that the film created and also to review scientific theories and interpretations to enhance our understanding. A strong focus will also be on interventions to assist these individuals in living more productive and fulfilling lives.

HISTORY

The terms Asperger Syndrome and high functioning autism have their origins in 1943 and 1944, when the seminal papers by Leo Kanner and Hans Asperger were first published. Although they never met, Asperger and Kanner had much in common. They were both born in Austria and trained in Vienna. Kanner was born in 1906, 10 years before Asperger. Kanner came to the United States in 1924 and eventually became head of the Child Psychiatric Clinic at Johns Hopkins University. Asperger remained in Vienna and became Chair of Pediatrics at the University of Vienna. Both were popular and respected authors in their fields; Kanner is credited with founding a new discipline through his first textbook on Child Psychiatry.

Amazingly, within a year of one another, each published a paper describing a group of children they noted to be different from others they saw in their clinics. Both even proposed variations of Bleuler's term "autism" as a diagnostic label, although this term later became associated with the group Kanner described but not Asperger's children.

The name they suggested for these children is not the only similarity between the two groups. There were many others, especially difficulties with social relationships, communication, and narrow, repetitive behaviors and routines. There were also important differences; Asperger's group was less commonly delayed in speech, had more motor deficits, had a later onset of problems, and were all boys. Questions arose in those days and persist today as to whether these were two separate disorders or perhaps artifacts of differences in the authors' interests, clinical referrals, or cultural biases.

KANNER'S ORIGINAL PAPER

Leo Kanner's 1943 paper described 11 children from his Child Psychiatric Unit who were more similar to one another than to the typical referrals he received. Their commonalities were symptoms fitting into three categories: peculiar language, social isolation, and insistence on sameness. Kanner's initial description was remarkable. Based only on his own observations, since no other reference work was available, he was able to highlight the characteristics that today define autism. Specifically, he noted social difficulties, communication problems, and repetitive and restricted activities (the so-called "triad of impairments" as they were labeled by Wing & Gould in 1979). Kanner viewed the social deficit as primary and chose the name "autism" as a way of highlighting this central feature of the disability.

Kanner distinguished autism from the childhood schizophrenia he typically saw in his clinic in several ways. He noted that people with schizophrenia withdrew from social relationships while children with autism never developed them in the first place: "There is from the start an extreme autistic aloneness that, whenever possible, disregards, ignores, shuts out anything that comes to the child from the outside" (1943, p. 242). He also noted the idiosyncratic features of language that were much more characteristic of autism than of schizophrenia. Kanner was fascinated by echolalia, pronoun reversals, and the unique forms of expression that characterized his group. Although Kanner saw autism and schizophrenia as separate in children, he assumed that autism was the earliest form and a precursor of adult schizophrenia (Eisenberg & Kanner, 1956). This assertion has since been disproven (Rutter & Schopler, 1978).

Kanner's paper was widely read and extremely influential, unusual for a first paper on a disorder (Gillberg, 1989). The reason for this is unclear, but perhaps it is because so many professionals were seeing children with these characteristics but had no way of conceptualizing or classifying them. One problem that has resulted is that the misconceptions in the original paper have been hard to overcome. Even though Kanner's work was remarkably accurate for a first description based on only 11 cases, he did argue that the children were mostly of normal or higher than normal intelligence, with parents from the higher social classes, and without neurological impairments. He also asserted that social deficits were primary. Since Kanner's time the definition of autism has expanded and some of these proposals have been refuted (see Mesibov et al., 1998). Many of his other ideas, however, are as accurate and relevant today as they were almost 60 years ago.

ASPERGER'S ORIGINAL PAPER

Asperger's paper (1944) was his doctoral thesis. Asperger's manuscript did not have the same impact as Kanner's, probably because it was published in German during World War II. Few English speakers had even heard of the paper before Lorna Wing's (1981) review of it almost 40 years later. From the available materials it seems as if Kanner was unaware of Asperger's work, although Asperger had read Kanner's and did, in fact, respond to his papers (Asperger, 1979).

Asperger's initial observations of these children were made during summer camp programs on his ward (Frith, 1991). During these activities Asperger noticed that some of the children did not fit in with the rest of the group, preferring to play alone and avoiding rough and tumble games. Asperger was concerned about these children and he set out to discover why and how they were different from the other children on the ward. With precision and empathy, Asperger described four boys and used the label "autistic psychopathy." This label has also been translated as "autistic personality disorder," which reflects Asperger's view of this syndrome as a stable personality trait present from birth, rather than a psychotic process.

Asperger described many different characteristics in his original paper. Like Kanner's, his observations were interesting, thought-provoking, and vivid. Unlike Kanner, however, Asperger did not articulate which of the characteristics he thought were essential for diagnosis, and which were not. Asperger's description reads like a detailed account of many common features he noted in the children, rather than a diagnostic description and analysis. Asperger never clarified if he thought the primary feature in his children was a disturbance in social contact. He noted only one linguistic peculiarity, which involved pragmatic language deficits (problems with using language functionally and appropriately). He interpreted the pragmatic language difficulties as he interpreted problems with eye gaze; these were seen as part of a fundamental disturbance in the expressive behaviors needed for social interaction. Asperger described the children he observed as unequal partners in social interactions, who were unable to interpret complex social cues. Asperger also noted the repetitive activities emphasized by Kanner. He saw them as another way the children used to follow their own interests and preoccupations at the expense of interacting, contacting, and learning from others.

Asperger placed greatest emphasis on one feature of his syndrome, which he termed "autistic intelligence." He viewed this as a form of independence and originality in thought which the children displayed, especially at school. This feature was both a strength and a weakness according to Asperger. Unlike other children who struggled to progress from mechanical learning to original thought, children with AS were capable only of forming their own strategies. They could not, or did not, follow those used by their teachers. To Asperger, this tendency reflected an intellectual strength, but also a lack of contact with those who tried to help them.

One example was a patient of Asperger's, Harro. Harro solved the problem "47 − 15" in this way: "Either add 3 and also 3 to that which should be taken away, or first take away 7 and then 8" (Asperger, 1991, p. 55). The method was so indirect that it often led to errors. This cumbersome and often impractical approach to problems, combined with difficulties in groups, was Asperger's explanation for the school difficulties so many of these children had in spite of average intelligence. Asperger recommended instruction in very basic and elementary academic skills and strategies, rather than allowing the children to use the faulty strategies they created on their own.

Although school difficulties were a concern, a more positive characteristic was the way these children channeled their intelligence and original thought into certain specific interests. Virtually all of Asperger's children had all-consuming interests in topics like chemistry, machinery, or space travel. Narrow in focus, these interests consumed a great deal of their time and energy.

Asperger's descriptions of their interests were accompanied by discussions of what he viewed as the negative aspect of their intelligence, "autistic acts of malice." Asperger interpreted some of the aberrant behaviors he observed as cunning uses of intelligence for malicious ends. For example, Asperger explained that Fritz deliberately misbehaved in his class because he enjoyed seeing his teacher become angry. Dewey (1991) has asserted that Asperger misinterpreted the intense pursuit of interests and lack of social understanding as malicious rather than oblivious. Asperger later modified his theory, stating that the children could not know how much they hurt other people, physically or emotionally.

SIMILARITIES BETWEEN KANNER AND ASPERGER

Both Asperger and Kanner noted symptoms falling into each of the three areas of the triad of impairment: social difficulties, communication problems, and repetitive and restricted activities. Both authors also took care to separate the children they described from those diagnosed with childhood schizophrenia. Although their interpretations were different, both noted that the parents of these children shared some of their behavioral features. Kanner's interpretation was that the parents' intellectual and cold demeanors may have caused their children to withdraw socially, contributing to their autism. This theory was later dismissed as evidence mounted that parents' behavior was not the cause of autism. Asperger saw parental behavior as evidence for a genetic phenotype. Asperger was also more aware of the social value of these characteristics; he noted that many of the parents were quite successful.

Both Kanner and Asperger also observed more males than females with these symptoms. In fact, Asperger originally thought that the syndrome existed only in males, a view he later reversed (Wing, 1981). Another feature noted by both authors was the clumsiness of the youngsters. Kanner mentioned it as an aside, while Asperger gave it a more central place as a defining characteristic. Today clumsiness is thought by some to be an important distinguishing feature between AS and HFA. Both Kanner and Asperger placed great emphasis on their clients' strengths and positive characteristics, frequently noting their special skills, absorbing interests, and strong rote memories.

BIASES, CULTURAL NORMS, AND REFERRAL SAMPLES

Although the similarities between the Kanner and Asperger descriptions are compelling, there were also some significant differences in their descriptions of the two groups. Before examining these differences in detail, it is important to acknowledge the strong cultural differences between the United States and Austria during the early 1940s, in order to separate cultural factors from actual differences between the children they were describing.

The most important cultural difference between the two countries was the influence of the Nazi Party in Vienna at the time of Asperger's work. Frith (1991) reported that Asperger's work was treated lightly in Austria because he was not a party activist. Also, Asperger was describing children with social problems in an environment where it could have been life-threatening to differ from the party ideal. Asperger was undoubtedly protective of his clients, so it is conceivable that he overemphasized the social value of their symptoms in order to protect the children. For example, he asserted that the children showed, "... a predestination for a particular profession from earliest youth. A particular line of work often grows naturally out of their special abilities .... A good professional attitude involves single-mindedness as well as the decision to give up a large number of other interests" (Asperger, 1991, pp. 88–89). Even though this emphasis on strengths might have been extreme and overstated, it represents a pleasant contrast to other psychiatric writings of that time which ignored positive qualities while overemphasizing weaknesses.

In terms of etiology and underlying deficits, the two authors seemed inclined to apply theories supported by their professional communities. Kanner was surrounded by proponents of psychodynamic theory. This could help explain Kanner's examination of parental characteristics and his misconception that autism was a reaction to parental rejection. His initial articles were followed by considerable psychodynamic theorizing on the etiology of autism (Bettleheim, 1967). It is fortunate, and a tribute to Kanner's scientific openness, that later scrutiny led him to reject this psychodynamic interpretation.

Asperger's work, on the other hand, did not have strong psychodynamic influences, despite Freud's early popularity in Vienna. By the time Asperger's thesis was published, Freud had left the country. Frith (1991) reports that Asperger's mentor, Lazar, formerly had employed a child psychoanalyst but later turned away from the theory, pronouncing it as inappropriate for children. Asperger must have concurred, as he considered AS genetic and did not even suggest psychodynamic or other environmental explanations.

Referral biases are also probable. Both authors worked with samples of children that were biased toward the higher end of the socioeconomic scale. In both countries in the 1940s, few families with limited economic resources sought psychiatric help. For this reason, highly successful and intelligent families were over-represented in psychiatric clinics. Therefore, both Kanner and Asperger overestimated the average economic and educational levels of families of children with AS/HFA.

Another referral bias, however, might have affected the authors differentially. Because Kanner's clinic focused on childhood schizophrenia, most of his referrals were initially thought to be schizophrenic, which suggests that they had the language skills to express unusual thoughts and perceptions. Thus, his original description of autism was based on this relatively high functioning group, which could explain his impression that children with autism have average intelligence. Asperger, on the other hand, had a reputation for helping children with disruptive behavior problems, and was most likely to see these types of children (Dewey, 1991). Those AS children who did not disrupt their classrooms were probably referred to other doctors in Austria, or perhaps not referred at all. Similarly, Frith (1991) suggested that during the 1940s, Austrians in general were more preoccupied with discipline than were Americans, and thus Asperger paid more attention to misbehavior. This could account for a higher incidence of mischief and malice in his AS students, which far exceeds the reports of any other investigator either during the period when Asperger wrote or afterwards.

DIFFERENCES BETWEEN KANNER'S AND ASPERGER'S DESCRIPTIONS

Beyond these potential biases lie further substantive differences between the two groups. Some of these may simply reflect the samples that each investigator selected but others may be keys to the differential diagnosis of separate disorders. In general, Asperger's clients were not as impaired as those of Kanner. Asperger's group was older by the time he saw them, and their communication problems seemed less severe. All of Asperger's patients were verbal but some of Kanner's were not. Also the Asperger children had less severe impairments in adaptive functioning, did better at school, and were less restricted in their activities.

The language in the Asperger group was more odd than impaired. He described his children as speaking like "little adults," in a pedantic manner using a large vocabulary. Kanner noted the extreme literalness in the children he saw who did speak. Social impairments in Asperger Syndrome were also less severe. All of the differences described to this point could merely be a function of the level of impairment, with the Kanner group being more impaired overall than the Asperger group.

There are, however, some differences between the two groups which cannot be explained simply on the basis of differences in overall functioning level. Kanner emphasized his patients' impaired relationships to people despite intact relationships to objects. Asperger saw both relationships as impaired. Asperger noted that his group collected objects just to possess them, rather than to make something out of them, change them, or play with them. Asperger also noted attention problems in his patients. Unlike impulsive and distractible children he had worked with, the children in this group attended to their own cues, rather than cues highlighted by teachers and parents. These attention problems caused school difficulties, even when Asperger's children had average or above intelligence.

These factors of attention differences and interest in collecting objects could have represented substantial differences between the groups. It is also possible, however, that Asperger made note of these characteristics while Kanner did not focus on them. Currently the controversy continues and there is not yet consensus on whether the groups are actually different or not.

OTHER NAMES FOR SIMILAR GROUPS

Before Asperger's seminal work, people with similar traits were described and discussed in the psychiatric literature under various names. Kretschmer (1925) included several Asperger-like symptoms in the case descriptions he used to categorize psychiatric patients into types. One form of "schizothymic" personality, which he called the "world-hostile idealist," was described as clinging rigidly to a favorite idea or "calling." This characteristic resembles the narrow interests of AS. Kretschmar also noted that this group was shy and awkward, only having friends who would participate in their interests.

Robinson and Vitale (1954) described three children with "circumscribed interest patterns." They placed such heavy emphasis on this one symptom that they believed it was the basis for a disorder in its own right. The children they described had significant social impairments but, unlike Kanner and Asperger, these authors believed that the social problems were secondary to the children's all-absorbing interests. The children became so absorbed in their interests that their social curiosity disappeared. These narrow interests were pursued to the exclusion of everything else.

Robinson and Vitale acknowledged the similarity of their group of children to those with autism. They believed they were different, however, in several important ways. First, they lacked an early emotional unresponsiveness that is typically seen in autism. These children seemed to have been normally-developing babies. At the time of referral, they were less withdrawn than children with autism, and showed less sameness-seeking behavior. Kanner wrote a response to the Robinson and Vitale article, concurring with the authors. He endorsed their differentiating factors and predicted that circumscribed interest patterns would become a separate diagnostic category. Actually, Robinson and Vitale's group sounds very similar to what we now call Asperger Syndrome.

Adams (1973) discussed Robinson and Vitale's group and their interests. He placed them on his "obsessive spectrum," and called their interests "impulsions." Emphasizing that these were different from compulsions, he went on to explain how impulsions were egodystonic. That means the clients displaying the symptoms had some awareness of how nonproductive and distracting they could be. Adams' cases would probably now be diagnosed with Obsessive–Compulsive Disorder (OCD). Adams' placement of children with special interests on the same spectrum with children with OCD, however, suggests that some of his cases actually had AS. Many of the symptoms he mentioned are consistent with AS: lack of spontaneity, poor motor coordination, social awkwardness and eccentricity, solitariness, and pedantic and literal speech.

In a book on learning and attention disorders, Kinsbourne and Caplan (1979) differentiated the "overfocused child" from impulsive children. While both groups had attention problems, the overfocused children were overly attentive to one particular topic to the exclusion of all others. The impulsive children, on the other hand, were simply very distractible, especially in school. Kinsbourne and Caplan also noted other characteristics of these overfocused children, including narrow interests, precision, not knowing when their work was finished, shyness, solitariness, sensitivity to criticism, formal speech, gaze avoidance, and stereotypies in times of distress. These symptoms are all common in both HFA and AS. The authors stated that these children were by no means autistic, but had many symptoms reminiscent of autism, although to a lesser degree of severity. The children's impairments were not considered severe enough to warrant a psychiatric diagnosis but the authors conceptualized a continuum including both over-focused children and those with autism.

One early diagnosis is still used by some workers. Since 1964, Sula Wolff has been studying a group of patients diagnosed with "schizoid personality disorder." During her earliest presentation of her work, Wolff was unfamiliar with Asperger's paper and description of his patients (Wolff & Barlow, 1979). After reading Asperger's work, she asserted that her group was almost identical to his except for two important differences: some of Wolff's clients were female and some developed schizophrenia in adulthood (Wolff & Chick, 1980). She acknowledged that her group indeed had symptoms of autism, but suggested that their degree of impairment was less severe. Wolff chose the term "schizoid personality disorder" for three reasons: (1) the condition was common and permanent; (2) the pattern was unchanging, fitting the definition of a personality disorder rather than an illness; and (3) the adult diagnostic category of schizoid personality disorder was comparable to what she saw in her children. Although the relationship between schizoid personality disorder and AS is still in dispute, Wolff's work has clearly demonstrated that their categories overlap significantly, and might actually be identical.

ASPERGER SYNDROME BEFORE WING'S PAPER

Lorna Wing, a British psychiatrist, is generally credited with introducing Asperger's work to the English-speaking autism community in 1981, in an important paper in which she reviewed Asperger's description, then added her own perspectives and clinical examples. However, years earlier Van Krevelen and Kuipers had mentioned Asperger in their 1962 article in English, and in 1971, Van Krevelen had written a paper about autism and AS. These papers, however, did not create the interest that followed Wing's later description. The problem was probably their early dates of publication, since autism had not yet been included in the DSM, the major classification system of psychiatric disorders, and there was not yet an active debate about diagnostic precision in autism. Also, these articles were published in child-focused journals, which limited their circulation. The greatest interest in Wing's article came from psychiatrists working with adults.

In his 1971 article, Van Krevelen directly compared autism and AS, which was still called "autistic psychopathy." He proposed four main differences between the disorders: (1) The onset of autism was in the first month and the onset of AS was not until the third year or even later; (2) Children with autism walked before talking but Asperger children talked before they walked. Also many children with autism were mute or had severe language delays and children with AS communicated well but one-sidedly; (3) Children with autism had poor eye contact because they were oblivious to others and children with AS avoided eye contact but participated in the world on their own terms; and (4) Autism was a psychotic process with a poor prognosis and AS was a personality trait with a much better prognosis.

These proposed differences reflect some of the misconceptions of those times about autism. For example, autism is no longer considered a psychotic process. Also, the description of AS was altered by Van Krevelen. Asperger did not set the age of onset at age 3 years but rather at 2 years or earlier. He did not interpret the poor eye contact as an aversion but rather as a result of treating people and objects similarly. Also, he thought that poor eye contact resulted from the inability of AS children to understand the communicative value of eye contact. Wing (1981) also noted that in real life symptoms are not as clear-cut as Van Krevelen described.

Although Van Krevelen's proposed differences have not survived in their present form, they have still contributed to the current conceptualization of the disorders. Another valuable contribution was Van Krevelen's description of two children in the same family, one with autism and the other with AS. The children's father also had Asperger-like symptoms. Van Krevelen proposed that AS was transmitted genetically through the father and that the children with autism would have had AS were it not for unspecified organic factors. Other authors have made this same point in subsequent years. For example, Burgoine and

Wing (1983) described a set of identical triplets who had AS. They noted that the brother with the most severe impairments had the most peri-natal and early childhood medical problems. Although they emphasized that the etiologic pathway could not be as simple as Van Krevelen's description, they concluded that the case study suggested that early severe brain damage can affect the way the condition is manifested. This early connection between brain damage from an insult and genetic factors as causes of autism, separately or in combination, is consistent with current thinking.

Bosch (1970) made another point that remains relevant today. In describing "autistic psychopathy," Bosch asserts that the difference between AS and autism is a matter of degree, and that the same person can be diagnosed with each disorder at different points in life. Bosch asserts that many people with AS would have been diagnosed with autism if they had been seen at younger ages. Likewise, some of his patients with autism improved enough with age to be indistinguishable from his adult clients with AS. The possibility of different diagnoses at different ages is still discussed today, though is not adequately reflected in any of the diagnostic systems.

WING'S CONTRIBUTIONS

Although the contributions reviewed in this chapter have had an important impact, Lorna Wing's (1981) paper was the major work to stimulate further review of Asperger's description and its relationship to that of Kanner. Even prior to her seminal article, Wing had described children with autistic features who did not fit Kanner's definition of autism precisely, but who were similar and could benefit from the same services (Wing, 1976). She described the work of Asperger and Van Krevelen and differentiated their groups from children with autism. Wing estimated that Kanner's definition only applied to 10% of children with autism, and she called attention to the need for new diagnoses or a broader definition of the disorder. In a 1979 community prevalence study, Wing and Gould found a "general impairment of reciprocal interaction" to be much more common than autism.

Wing (1986) wrote her 1981 article partially in response to Wolff and Barlow (1979). She disagreed with their classification of AS as a personality disorder, instead viewing it as a developmental problem on the autistic spectrum. The paper reflected Wing's desire for a broader conceptualization of autism. She described Asperger's cases, as well as her own, and changed the disorder's name from "autistic psychopathy" to "Asperger's Syndrome." Wing reasoned that the term "psychopathy" was too often associated with anti-social behavior and could cause too much confusion. Wing also included girls among her cases, arguing that although AS was more common in males, it clearly could occur in females as well.

In addition to changing the name and including girls, Wing made other modifications in the definition of the disorder. First she high-lighted aspects of developmental history that Asperger had not mentioned. She noted that before one year of age children with AS showed little interest or pleasure in social contact, limited babbling, and no joint attention. An example was if a child saw an interesting toy in the store he would not demand a parent's attention by pointing to it. Normally developing children, in contrast, have an "intense urge to communicate" before the development of speech, according to Wing. Wing also noted that some children with AS had no pretend play. Those able to pretend confined their play to a few set themes, often enacting scenes repetitively. These children did not involve others in their play, unless the other children followed commands and allowed the child with AS to dominate the scene.

Another modification was Wing's assertion that children with AS did not necessarily excel in language as Asperger originally claimed. Her patients eventually developed good grammar and a large vocabulary, but the content of their speech was impaired and much of it was copied from other people or from books. To Wing, it seemed as if they had learned language by rote. Her patients often knew difficult words but not easier ones. There was also a pronounced impairment in nonverbal communication. Wing examined motor and language milestones noting that fewer than half of her patients walked at the usual age and many were slow talkers. These observations refuted Asperger's and Van Krevelen's belief that children with AS talked before they walked. They are also inconsistent with the current DSM-IV definition (to be discussed in Chapter 2) that emphasizes normal language development.

As noted previously, Asperger emphasized his clients' originality and creativity in their chosen fields. Wing modified this to a more measured view of the skills and interests in AS. She noted that her patients often selected an unusual aspect of a commonly interesting topic, rendering the topic somewhat inappropriate. She described their pursuit of interests as "narrow, pedantic, literal, but logical" (p. 118). Rather than an indication of unusually high intelligence, the interests and special skills were largely based on rote memory. Understanding of meaning was universally poor. Wing did not dismiss Asperger's rosier view of interests completely, however, since she noted that her patients were more severely impaired than Asperger's.

Wing's final modification involved the prognosis of people with AS. She emphasized that it was possible to have both AS and mental retardation. Because not all people with AS were of normal or high intelligence, Wing insisted that the generally accepted notions about the disorder's prognosis needed to be altered to reflect variations in intelligence levels. Also, comorbid psychiatric disorders often affected the prognosis. Depression and anxiety were common, and Wing surmised this was because of these clients' increased awareness that they were different from others. This awareness typically came during adolescence or young adulthood.

Wing's documentation of poor prognoses and more comorbidity in her sample represents a broadening of Asperger's definition of AS to include lower functioning people. Disagreeing with Asperger, Van Krevelen, and Wolff, Wing concluded that, at the time of her writing, the available evidence pointed to a distinction between AS and autism based on severity. The other authors believed that there were fundamental differences in the nature of the disorders. Nevertheless, Wing advocated keeping the term AS, although she has reevaluated this position more recently and now questions whether a separate diagnosis of Asperger's Syndrome is really productive after all.

Following Wing's 1981 paper, there was an explosion of research attempting to clarify qualitative differences between HFA and AS. This issue has still not been settled and will be addressed in the next chapter on Diagnosis and Classification.

Wing (1986) has noted important sequelae from her paper. Referrals from adult psychiatrists, suspecting that their patients had AS, increased significantly. Unexpectedly, these included referrals from forensic psychiatrists who surmised that their patients had committed crimes because of their narrow interests and limited social understanding. These referrals helped Wing to gain more information about the clinical picture of AS in adulthood. The disadvantage of these cases for understanding AS was that they generally relied on retrospective reports of developmental histories. Such retrospective reports are notoriously unreliable and can often result in misdiagnoses and misperceptions of the developmental histories of disorders. Confusion based on retrospective reports is especially troubling in identifying whether a link exists between criminality and AS, which is still difficult to determine.

Another consequence of the Wing publication has been an expansion of the understanding of autism. Wing helped increase public awareness that the autism spectrum includes more than Kanner's initial definition. As a result of her work, misdiagnoses of higher functioning people with autism or AS have dramatically decreased.

OTHER EARLY REPORTS OF HIGHER FUNCTIONING AUTISM

Yirmiya and Sigman (1991) listed many of the early terms used for higher functioning autism: normally intelligent autistic, near-normal autistic, non-retarded autistic, higher-level autistic, high-IQ autistic, and relatively gifted children with Kanner-type autism. Because of the common stereotype of autism as a disorder resulting in a very low level of functioning, many people with higher functioning autism were misdiagnosed with learning disabilities, hyperactivity, obsessive–compulsive disorder, and related conditions. It was hard for parents and professionals to believe that verbal children of average intelligence could have autism.

An early article by two parents, Dewey and Everard (1974), provided a clear description of autism in a higher functioning individual. They described common manifestations of each area of the triad in "the near normal autistic adolescent." Dewey and Everard cautioned that even though these higher functioning children had better prognoses, they still had significant impairments in all three areas of the triad, and required intensive and long-term interventions. Based on their personal experiences as parents, they provided advice about how to use interests and talents to the advantage of people with HFA.

Bartak and Rutter (1976) also contributed much to our early understanding of HFA by clearly differentiating it from lower functioning autism. In a study of 36 children (17 with nonverbal IQ's <69 and 19 with nonverbal IQ's of 70 or above), they reported significant differences between the groups in terms of a number of variables. As a group, the higher-functioning children had:

- less impaired responsiveness in infancy
- better cooperative play and emotional expressiveness
- fewer unusual social interactions
- more rituals but less resistance to change and attachment to odd objects
- less self-injurious behavior
- fewer hand stereotypies

Also, in this group the average age for first use of single words was 2 years 6 months, and average age for first use of phrase speech was 4 years 8 months.

--- THE ROLE OF THE DSM

In the United States, the most widely used definitions of autism and AS are contained in the current edition of the Diagnostic and Statistical Manual of Mental Disorders, called DSM-IV, which is published by the American Psychiaric Association (APA, 1994). The first DSM was published in 1952, with revisions in 1968, 1980, 1987, and 1994.

Autism appeared for the first time in the DSM-III (APA, 1980). This first official definition did not, however, reflect the disorder's heterogeneity. Many higher functioning people with autism did not meet the narrowly defined diagnosis, and thus were diagnosed with "Infantile autism, residual state," indicating that the symptoms were no longer present. As a result they were disqualified from services under the mistaken impression that they had "recovered" from autism. Because of its inadequacies, the DSM-III definition played a large role in the development of the AS diagnosis, by making it clear that a diagnostic label was needed for adults with higher-functioning autism to reflect their life-long disability. Wing (1986) suggested retaining the strict DSM-III definition and including AS as a new label within the autism spectrum. This is what occurred in DSM-IV (1994). In between these two editions, however, came DSM-III-R (1987), which simply broadened the 1980 definition of autism so that many of those who had been excluded previously would now meet the criteria.

AS was included in the DSM-IV series for the first time in 1994 (the DSM-IV) using the term "Asperger's Disorder." The DSM-IV has recently undergone a text revision in several sections, including the section that includes autism and AS. Additional examples and descriptions are being added, although the specific diagnostic criteria are not being changed.

SUMMARY AND CONCLUSION

Beginning in the early 1940s and continuing to the present, studies of HFA and AS have increased our understanding in a parallel fashion to the development of knowledge in the field of autism in general. Although they were not familiar with one another's work, Kanner and Asperger described many similar and overlapping characteristics. Later investigations analyzed similarities and differences between these descriptions and also have looked at the overlap between both of them and related conditions like schizoid personality disorders or learning and attention problems. The work of Lorna Wing in the 1980s has been instrumental in highlighting AS and its relationship to high functioning autism.

Current researchers continue to build on the strong foundation that has been provided. The result has been a dramatic increase in our understanding of high functioning people with autism. The distinction between autism and AS, however, remains unclear and unresolved. Current research continues to focus on the question of whether HFA and AS should be considered as separate conditions. With this historical background, we will turn to what has been learned about the people who have been identified with these conditions.

Diagnosis and Classification

By the time Sammy Wilson was 11 years old, his parents had filled two loose-leaf notebooks with reports from evaluation centers, therapists, and doctors. While the various professionals had been kind, thorough, and skilled in their evaluations, each one had used a different diagnosis or label, and Sammy's parents remained confused about what his problem really was. As a young child, he had been considered somewhat "oppositional" and "defiant." Later, the possibility of Attention Deficit/Hyperactivity Disorder was raised. In school, he received special education resource help in written language under the label of Learning Disability, but Mr. and Mrs. Wilson's other son had a learning disability also, and it was clear to them that Sammy was different. He didn't have any real friends, and he spent most of his free time looking at catalogues of laboratory equipment. Recently they had read an article about autism, but while parts of the description sounded like Sammy, the Wilsons couldn't believe that such a serious diagnosis could apply to Sammy, who had just been recommended for a summer honors program in science. He seemed far too capable to have a disability, yet something was clearly wrong. It was very frustrating not to have a name or an explanation for his difficulties.

INTRODUCTION

Diagnosis in psychiatry and psychology is very different from diagnosis in internal medicine or pediatrics. As Szatmari (2000) has pointed out, a person does not "have" autism in the same way he might "have" strep throat. Medical diagnoses can generally be confirmed by specific laboratory tests with tightly defined values for normal, borderline, and abnormal findings (such as blood sugar level, blood pressure, lung function, etc.). But in developmental and behavioral disorders, diagnosis refers to global patterns of functioning, which are much more difficult to define and measure, and which may vary along several dimensions, including over time (particularly in childhood) and in different situations (such as the quiet home of an only child vs. a large, noisy school cafeteria). The more multi-faceted the disorder, the more difficult it is to develop precise diagnostic criteria. As Lorna Wing eloquently wrote, "Recognizing patterns within this bewildering complexity is akin to classifying clouds" (1998, p. 11).

Within the autism spectrum, more capable or higher functioning people with Asperger Syndrome (AS) or autism are among the most difficult to diagnose. Although they might show the same difficulties as more handicapped people with autism in the triad of impairments (social interaction, communication, and restricted patterns of behavior; Wing & Gould, 1979), these deficits are usually more subtle and can be difficult to identify. For example, higher functioning people with autism or AS might engage in social behavior but it might not be as reciprocal as one sees in normally developing people, or their ability to make friends might be more limited. Language skills can be well developed but there might be a problem with turn-taking in conversations. Also, people with AS/HFA often have pedantic speech, using awkward phrases and big words. Their narrow interests are sometimes harder to identify than the repetitive, self-stimulatory behaviors often observed in more impaired people with autism. Narrow interests might include preoccupation with thoughts or facts such as numerical combinations, birthdays, train schedules, a time in history, cash registers, or dinosaurs.

As we have seen, Leo Kanner and Hans Asperger took on the task of describing these behaviors, writing papers labeling the pattern of "autism" among children they worked with. Over the past 50 years, other professionals in the field also wrote descriptive papers, shared observations at conferences, and met to develop consensus statements regarding diagnostic criteria. The two major diagnostic systems currently in use are the ICD-10 (International Classification of Diseases – Tenth Edition; World Health Organization, 1993) and the DSM-IV (Diagnostic and Statistical Manual of Mental Disorders – Fourth Edition; American Psychiatric Association, 1994). The ICD-10, as its name implies, has been developed and used internationally to categorize both medical and psychiatric/developmental disorders, while the DSM-IV was developed in the United States and is more narrowly focused on psychiatric and related conditions. In terms of autism and AS, the ICD-10 and DSM-IV definitions are closely coordinated. Since the DSM-IV is more widely used for clinical purposes in this country, we will focus on its criteria and description of autism and AS.

The section of the DSM-IV concerned with autism spectrum disorders contains specific criteria in each of three areas of impairment: social interactions, verbal and nonverbal communication, and unusual behavior and interests. Each of these three areas contains four criteria, for a total of twelve. The social and behavior/interests criteria for autism and AS are identical, while there are no criteria related to impaired communication in AS; in fact, some elements of communication development are required to be normal. For a diagnosis of autism, at least six of the twelve criteria must be met (at least two in the social area and at least one each in the communication and behavior/interest areas). For a diagnosis of Asperger Syndrome, at least two social criteria and at least one of the behavior/interests criteria must be met. Following are the areas of overlap in DSM-IV between autism and Asperger Syndrome.

COMMON ELEMENTS IN DSM-IV CRITERIA FOR ASPERGER SYNDROME AND AUTISM

Qualitative Impairment in Reciprocal Social Interaction

Note that "impairment" does not mean that the skill or behavior is totally absent, but that it is limited or unusual in some way, compared to typical people. Also, the specific manifestations of AS might be more subtle or require more cognitive skills than behaviors characteristic of autism that meet the same criteria.

The first aspect of the social criterion is "marked impairment in the use of multiple nonverbal behavior such as eye-to-eye gaze, facial expression, body postures, and gestures to regulate social interaction." Examples of behaviors meeting this criterion would be either avoiding eye contact or staring too intently at another person's face, having a flat facial expression or constantly smiling, or limited use of typical gestures such as head nodding, pointing, or shrugging the shoulders.

The second element of the social criterion is "failure to develop peer relationships appropriate to one's developmental level." This lack of friends can occur for several reasons. Some children with autism/AS are simply not interested in having friends, apparently finding social relationships too confusing or unpredictable. Others might want friends but not understand how to go about establishing these relationships. For example, at younger ages they might hug, pinch, or push other children in an attempt to establish social contact. Older, higher-functioning youngsters might attempt to talk with peers, but choose topics that are not interesting to the other person. Some people with AS/HFA, especially during adolescence, become depressed by their inability to establish friendships. Other individuals might naively believe that all of the members of their class are their friends. Virtually all people with autism/AS have difficulty comprehending fully what it means to be someone's friend.

It is important to remember that the definition of this social deficit involves peer relationships relative to the individual's developmental level. So, for example, a person with severe mental retardation and a mental age of 2–3 years who participates in parallel play next to another child is exhibiting friendship skills at an appropriate developmental level. However, a 10-year-old with intact intellectual skills who participates in parallel play but is unable to name a single best friend is not at an appropriate developmental level.

"A lack of spontaneous seeking to share enjoyment, interests, or achievements with other people" is a third aspect of this social criterion. A child with autism/AS, might, for example, become very excited when he hears certain TV commercials, sees favorite objects, or reaches an advanced level on a computer game, yet not try to call anyone's attention to these experiences. Normally developing children are typically very motivated to seek attention and show objects of interest to their parents and others, in order to share their pleasure. The absence of these behaviors, often called "joint attention", is one of the earliest symptoms of autism.

The final element in the social area is "lack of social or emotional reciprocity." This means that people with autism/AS have difficulty with the give and take of social and feeling-oriented interactions with other people. While many people with autism and AS are interested in some type of social interaction, they generally have trouble monitoring and maintaining these interactions. That is, it is difficult for them to focus simultaneously on what they are thinking, what they want to say next, and how the other person is reacting and thinking. As a result, they appear socially insensitive or even uninterested. For example, a child with autism or AS might not understand the social excitement of a classmate who is describing a wonderful weekend, and so might fail to respond, or change the topic, or walk away abruptly. Other individuals may monopolize conversations talking about their special interests, without realizing that listeners are bored or in a hurry and without soliciting their input, thus appearing odd, self-absorbed, or boring.

Restricted Repetitive and Stereotyped Patterns of Behavior, Interests, and Activities

This diagnostic criterion involves clearly unusual behavior, rather than impaired or limited skills. For both autism and AS, at least one of the following four elements of the criterion is required for DSM-IV diagnosis.

First among these is "encompassing preoccupation with one or more stereotyped and restricted patterns of interest that is abnormal either in intensity or focus." In lower-functioning autism, examples of this symptom are playing exclusively with one object, often an unusual object (such as string, sticks, rubber glove, or pantyhose), or playing with toys in an unusual way (such as lining up or spinning all objects). Among older, higher-functioning people with autism or AS, this symptom is often seen as learning vast amounts of information about highly restricted topics, such as weather maps, highways, zip codes, sports statistics, etc.

The second element of this criterion is "apparently inflexible adherence to specific, nonfunctional routines or rituals." For example, children with autism might tantrum unless specific bedroom routines are followed in precise order, sit only in a particular place in the car, or demand that their food be served in a particular way (such as eating a sandwich only if it is cut diagonally). A child with autism might also become agitated if a parent deviates from an expected driving route or the mailman knocks at the side door rather than ringing the front doorbell. Even high functioning adults can become agitated in unpredictable situations or when their routines are changed or their expectations are not met.

"Stereotyped and repetitive motor mannerisms" is the third symptom of this criterion. Behaviors such as body rocking, hand flapping, spinning, and head banging are most commonly seen among younger and lower functioning children. Even higher functioning adults, however, might flap their hands or hop excitedly when something exciting or important is happening.

A final manifestation of this criterion in this group is "persistent preoccupation with parts of objects." This is among the most frequently observed characteristics of autism. Children with autism might smell their toys, spin the wheels of their truck, slam doors repeatedly, or be obsessed by small visual details, such as strings on clothing, dirt on window panes, slightly open drawers. Higher-functioning individuals might over-focus on thinking about certain small elements of their world, such as mathematical calculations or the makes of cars driven by everyone they know. This preoccupation with parts of objects and details sometimes interferes with the person's ability to understand the larger meaning of the various aspects of the environment.

PRIMARY DIFFERENCE IN DSM-IV CRITERIA FOR ASPERGER SYNDROME AND AUTISM

As we have described, identical criteria of social deficits and restricted interests are used to diagnose both autism and AS. Autism involves a third diagnostic criterion, "Qualitative Impairments in Communication." This criterion has four elements, at least one of which must be present for the diagnosis of autism. These four elements are (1) delays in or total lack of the development of language; (2) impairment in initiation of language or sustaining conversations with others; (3) stereotypic, repetitive use of language; and (4) lack of spontaneous, make-believe play.

In contrast, for AS the criterion of impaired communication is not present. On the contrary, a diagnostic criterion for AS according to DSM-IV is that "there is no clinically significant general delay in language," defined as developing single words by the age of two years and using phrases for communication by the age of three years.

Based on the historical perspective presented in Chapter 1, it is immediately clear that the DSM-IV criteria represent marked changes and omissions from the concept of AS that evolved from Hans Asperger's work. The most important difference involves the issue of communication and language.

Asperger (1944) himself noted pragmatic language deficits in his students. He saw his students as having problems using language in typical ways, which he described as a fundamental disturbance in the expressive language characteristics that are necessary for social interaction. He also noted oddities in their language, describing his children as speaking like "little adults" in a pedantic manner using a large vocabulary. Van Krevelen (1971) also highlighted the one-sidedness and lack of reciprocity in the communication of children with AS. Similarly, as described in Chapter 1, Wing discussed various atypical features of the language and communication of children with AS.

More recently, Twachtman-Cullen (1998) has described the following difficulties with the DSM-IV criteria for AS: First, the DSM-IV definition uses the term "clinically significant general delay in language" which is open to different interpretations. Second, the milestone of single words at age two years, used as an example of normal language development, actually represents a significant expressive language delay. Third, use of "communicative phrases" at age three years involves not just saying a sequence of words but also communication, meaning the appropriate use of language for social purposes, which is very frequently not normal in youngsters with AS, even if they speak in phrases or sentences.

Another difficulty with the DSM-IV criterion of delayed language development is that it is becoming clear that empirical support is lacking for this as a differentiating factor between autism and AS.

A study (Szatmari et al., 1995) did find that 4–6 year old autistic children with delayed/deviant language had more social impairments and atypical behaviors than those with normal language development. However, a series of studies by Eisenmajer, Prior, and colleagues (1996, 1998) with high functioning individuals on the autism spectrum found that a history of early language delay did not predict eventual severity of autistic symptomatology; that is, by age 11 years there were no differences in autistic symptomatology between individuals with or without early language delay as defined by DSM-IV. Also, when the statistical technique of "cluster analysis" was used to identify subgroups of high-functioning autistic children, early language development variables were not useful in differentiating the groups. Similarly, Miller and Ozonoff (2000) reported that in a carefully diagnosed sample of youngsters with either HFA or AS, the history of normal early language development was not specific to AS, since it was also reported in 42% of the children with HFA.

Many research findings indicate that some aspects of the language of people with AS, such as the development of vocabulary and sentence structure, are indeed eventually fairly normal. However, there are often problems with other elements of communication, such as speech patterns (such as talking too quickly or too loud), using inappropriately pedantic speech or awkward phrases, misunderstanding idioms, humor, sarcasm, and other non-literal meanings of spoken language, talking too much and disregarding cues from the conversational partner, and having difficulty maintaining a conversation (Klin et al., 2000; Landa, 2000; Minshew et al., 1995).

In summary, the DSM-IV diagnostic criterion of unimpaired communication in AS is inconsistent with the clinical and research literature. Further, this section of DSM-IV sets out inaccurate developmental milestones and confounds language and communication.

ADDITIONAL ASPECTS OF AS IN DSM-IV

Three additional elements are included in DSM-IV for the diagnosis of AS:

A. "There is no clinically significant delay in cognitive development or in the development of age-appropriate self-help skills, adaptive behavior (other than in social interaction), and curiosity about the environment in childhood." This contrasts sharply with the criterion for autism of delays in social interaction, social language use, or symbolic/imaginative play before age 3 years.

Volkmar and Klin (1998) have pointed out that the wording of this criterion for AS is potentially misleading, since it can be interpreted as meaning that there are no significant adaptive behavior deficits and delays throughout the lifespan, while in fact such impairments are often seen in later years with AS. The equivalent criterion in ICD-10 is more clearly worded, indicating that only significant delays in adaptive behavior skills during the period of early development (to age 3 years) would exclude a diagnosis of AS.

B. "Criteria are not met for another specific Pervasive Developmental Disorder or Schizophrenia." The effect of this criterion is that if the individual meets criteria for autism, then autism would be diagnosed instead of AS.

Since we have seen that the social and behavioral descriptions of autism and AS are identical, this means that the decision between a diagnosis of autism or AS comes down to early developmental factors. By DSM-IV definition, early development in AS is essentially normal in the areas of language/communication, cognitive, adaptive and curiosity, while in autism, at least in terms of the latter three factors, it is not. (The DSM-IV does not have specific criteria regarding early language development milestones in autism.)

There are several potential problems with relying on information about early history to make the differential diagnosis. First, different aspects of developmental progress can be inconsistent: for example, first words spoken on time but phrase speech delayed; normal cognitive development but delayed adaptive/self-help skills (such as toilet training or eating with a fork). Second, retrospective information about developmental history is sometimes not available, and sometimes not very reliable. Third, as mentioned previously, criteria involving the phrase "clinically significant delay" are open to various interpretations. Ironically, Landa (2000) has pointed out, as more developmental screening and early intervention programs are developed, more standardized test scores are available for young children, often documenting delays or disorders that might otherwise have been overlooked until after the criterion age of 3 years. Fourth, as we have seen, the "normal language/communication" criterion is confusing. In spite of these various issues, based on current criteria it appears that any indication of delay prior to age 3 years should result in a diagnosis of autism rather than AS.

> C. "The disturbance causes clinically significant impairment in social, occupational, or other important areas of functioning." This means that slightly eccentric interests and awkward social skills that do not result in "significant impairment" would not lead to a diagnosis of AS. Again, this criterion involves subjective judgment about what constitutes "clinically significant" impairment.

Poor motor skills and motor planning difficulties are not formal criteria for AS in DSM-IV, although they are described in the narrative portion that accompanies the official list of symptoms. Asperger himself considered that his children were markedly clumsy, and some researchers think that poor motor skills are an important distinguishing feature between autism and AS. Many studies have confirmed that youngsters diagnosed with AS scored below average or more poorly than control groups on measures of motor development. However, while the clinical lore related to autistic children is that they are very agile and well-coordinated, a number of recent studies have found that motor delays and poor coordination are also very common in autistic children and adults (Ghaziuddin et al., 1994; Manjiviona & Prior, 1995; Miller & Ozonoff, 2000; Minshew et al., 1997; Rapin, 1996). There is no conclusive evidence that motor skill development differentiates autism from AS (Ozonoff & Griffith, 2000).

CURRENT PERSPECTIVES ON THE RELATIONSHIP OF AUTISM AND AS

In 1981, Lorna Wing introduced Asperger's work to the English-speaking world by describing his ideas then adding her own perspectives. In

1991, Uta Frith, another prominent researcher and clinician in the field, translated Asperger's paper into English and published it along with papers from other major scholars. And so for the past 10–20 years, English-speaking researchers and other professionals have lined up on different sides of the question, "Is there a meaningful difference between AS and HFA?" A fair number of them originally thought the answer was "yes," but have since changed their opinions. Interestingly, two psychologists have analyzed the descriptions of the four children Asperger described, and made the case that all of them would be diagnosed with autism rather than AS according to DSM-IV criteria (Miller & Ozonoff, 1997).

A recent study (Eisenmajer et al., 1996) compared the diagnoses used by community professionals (child psychiatrists, psychologists, and pediatricians) in Australia and England against early and current symptoms in a group of high functioning individuals. It was clear that many professionals had disregarded the official diagnostic criteria in the ICD-10 and DSM-IV, since 43% of the individuals diagnosed with AS had a history of delayed language onset, and 89% of them had a history of language disorder. It appeared that the professionals used the diagnosis of AS for individuals (1) with some social interests and (2) better (although not normal) current verbal skills. While these might be reasonable variables on which to differentiate various forms or degrees of autism, as we have seen they are not the variables on which the DSM-IV or ICD-10 rely.

Some of the major research groups looking at AS are those of Gillberg in Sweden, Szatmari in Canada, Ozonoff in Utah, Wing in England, and Volkmar, Klin, and Sparrow in Connecticut. Each of these groups has compared large numbers of individuals diagnosed with AS or autism. Unfortunately, until recently each research group has used a slightly different definition of AS, either because the work was done prior to DSM-IV/ICD-10, or because they disagreed with one or more elements of those diagnostic systems. As a result, it is not at all clear that the different researchers were studying the same phenomenon.

This is a particular problem when the question being studied was "Is AS meaningfully different from HFA?" It seems likely that some of the subjects described as having AS might easily have been diagnosed by someone else with HFA and vice versa. This would make differences between the two groups impossible to interpret, and would also mean that studies finding no differences between the diagnoses might be inaccurate.

At the present time, there is no professional consensus as to whether differences between AS and HFA are significant enough to justify the use of two diagnostic labels. The arguments for separate diagnoses are as follows:

1	People with AS have less atypical language and communication than people with HFA.
2	People with AS have more social interest and less unusual social behavior than people with HFA.
3	People with AS generally have Verbal IQs that are markedly higher than their Performance IQs, while the opposite pattern is true of people with HFA.
4	People with AS are more likely to have significant motor clumsiness and delayed development of motor skills than people with HFA.

The arguments against separate diagnoses are as follows:

1	Autism varies in severity and is associated with varying levels of intelligence. What is called AS is mild autism with average to above-average intelligence, associated with less impairment in all areas of functioning.
2	The differences seen between groups in research studies are tainted by methodological limitations, including inconsistent or evolving diagnostic criteria and possible circularity (that is, for example, groups were divided based on early language delay, then found to differ on current language skills).
3	The pattern of Verbal vs. Performance IQ is not specific to either group (see discussion of IQ test results in Chapter 3).
4	Research indicates significant levels of motor coordination difficulties in both groups.

Several recent studies and reviews of the neuropsychological research comparing AS and HFA (Manjiviona & Prior, 1999; Miller &

Ozonoff, 2000; Ozonoff & Griffith, 2000) have concluded that convincing empirical support in neuropsychology for the two separate diagnoses has not so far been established. Schopler (1994) has used the term "premature popularization" to describe the rapid and broad adoption of the concept of AS. However, this does not mean that the distinction will not and should not eventually be made. Ozonoff and Griffith (2000) state that "it would be as premature to rule out the validity of AS as it would be to treat it as an entity clearly distinguishable from classic autism" (p. 88).

In spite of the limited evidence for two separate disorders, many parents and professionals appear to be more comfortable with a diagnosis of AS than one of HFA. Wing (1986) noted that parents and professionals were more receptive if a clinician diagnosed a child with "an interesting condition called Asperger's Syndrome" rather than a form of autism. She suggested waiting to make the connection between AS and autism until later in treatment so that parents could have time to adjust to having a relatively palatable diagnosis, while eventually getting services and support from agencies serving the autistic population. Gillberg (1989) concurred, emphasizing that parents have no preconceived notions about the diagnosis of AS.

The wish to see AS as a separate disorder from autism is understandable, given many parents' view of autism as the worst possible diagnosis, connoting extreme impairment, social isolation, and bizarre behavior. There are other ways, however, to soften the blow of a diagnosis besides withholding the link to autism (Shea, 1984, 1993). Providing a picture to parents that is not totally complete in its information creates a number of other difficulties. Also, because AS is not yet widely known among the general public, it is much harder to obtain special education, vocational support services, and other forms of assistance that are directed toward people with recognized disabilities.

Perhaps as part of the desire to portray AS as a separate disorder from autism, some professionals and parents continue to return to the original papers of Kanner and Asperger, looking for details that would indicate that the two disorders are fundamentally different. However, it is not reasonable to expect that the initial descriptions and thoughts of early workers in the field of autism would be complete and accurate according to current research-based knowledge. Continuing to examine in minute detail the seminal articles of Kanner and Asperger is probably not a productive activity (Klin et al., 2000). What is important for our clients and their families today is what we now know, rather than what was thought in the early 1940s, brilliant and astute though that early thinking was.

DIAGNOSIS OF RELATED DISORDERS

Deciding between the diagnosis of HFA and AS is only one of several diagnostic dilemmas. Not only do AS and HFA overlap with one another, they also share symptoms with numerous other behavioral, psychiatric, and developmental disorders. In this section we will review the most common of the overlapping conditions.

The disorders most often considered along with AS/HFA include Obsessive–Compulsive Disorder, Nonverbal Learning Disability, Schizoid Personality Disorder, Semantic–Pragmatic Language Disorders, and Pervasive Developmental Disorder–Not Otherwise Specified.

Obsessive–Compulsive Disorder (OCD)

Obsessive–Compulsive disorder is characterized by repetitive thoughts and/or behaviors. A distinction is made between obsessions, which are "recurrent and persistent thoughts, impulses, or images" that are worrisome (DSM-IV, p. 422), and compulsions, which are non-functional repetitive behaviors or mental acts that are performed to reduce the anxiety from the obsession. An example of an obsession might be an ongoing concern about bacterial infections, resulting in the compulsion of continuous hand washing and cleaning. Compulsive behaviors can also take the form of a driven desire to behave according to rigid rules, such as always entering a room by the same door or always tapping the plate with a fork before each bite of food.

People with AS/HFA often display ritualistic, stereotypic, repetitive behaviors like those that characterize people with OCD. There are several points to consider in distinguishing Obsessive–Compulsive behaviors from AS/HFA.

First, the narrow interests associated with AS are not the same as the obsessive thoughts in OCD. Individuals with AS usually show an intense preoccupation with topics that they think and talk about repetitively. However, engagement in these interests tends to reduce their anxiety; in contrast, the obsessive thoughts in OCD cause anxiety. Also, the content of the repetitive thoughts in OCD is more likely to involve themes of aggression, contamination, sex, religion, bodily concerns, or symmetry; these topics are much less common in AS (Baron-Cohen & Wheelwright, 1999; McDougle et al., 1995). Further, most individuals with OCD recognize that their compulsive behaviors are unreasonable, while this level of insight is not characteristic of AS. Developmental histories can also be helpful in making these discriminations. People with OCD usually do not have a preschool or early childhood onset of their preoccupations and, in fact, usually have typical early developmental histories. Early developmental or social problems are much more often seen in AS or HFA, as is the co-existence of Tourette's Syndrome or epilepsy.

It is possible, however, for individuals to have both AS and OCD.

Semantic–Pragmatic Disorder

Semantic–Pragmatic Disorder (Bishop, 2000) is a developmental language disorder characterized by near-normal grammar, vocabulary and speech production, but impaired use of language in content and comprehension (that is, semantics) and function that is, pragmatic deficits). Children with this disorder have difficulty initiating and sustaining conversations, staying on topic, and using words in context, as do children with AS/HFA.

Children with Semantic–Pragmatic Disorder usually have delayed language milestones (Szatmari, 1998). Based on DSM-IV this differentiates them from children with AS, although we have already seen that the lack of language delays as a diagnostic criterion for AS is problematic.

A recent study (Gagnon et al., 1997) suggests that most children with this disorder also fit criteria for an autism spectrum disorder. Therefore, these authors question the value of Semantic–Pragmatic

Disorder as a separate diagnostic label. Some have argued that children going to language or communication clinics are likely to be given this label, particularly in the United Kingdom, while few other places use this diagnosis with any frequency.

Schizoid Personality Disorder

This disorder is characterized by "a pervasive pattern of detachment from social relationships and a restricted range of expression of emotions in interpersonal settings" (DSM-IV, p. 638). Thus, lack of empathy, limited social skills and friendships, social aloofness or apparent insensitivity, and single-mindedness are characteristics shared by people with AS and Schizoid Personality Disorder. Wolff (1998, 2000) and others have noted that central characteristics of Asperger Disorder are very similar to those observed in Schizoid Personality Disorder and argue that the two disorders should be classified together.

However, in the Schizoid Personality group, deficits in social interactions are often less severe than in AS/HFA and frequently are not apparent until later school years or early adulthood, instead of in preschool and early school years. Communication deviations are subtle and have a less profound effect on relationships in this group than is usually seen in children with AS/HFA. Imagination and fantasy are evident in this group, compared to the concreteness and severe creativity deficits seen in AS/HFA. Also, individuals with Schizoid Personality Disorder do not have the intense special interests of people with AS/HFA, and in fact rarely express strong interest or pleasure. Schizoid Personality Disorder appears to have a genetic link to schizophrenia, while AS/HFA does not. Schizoid children have increased rates of other psychiatric disorders as well. However, chances for occupational success and independent living are much greater in Schizoid Personality Disorder than in AS/HFA.

In spite of these differences, Wolff (1998) still argues that Schizoid Personality Disorder might be part of the autism spectrum. She urges more research and finer discriminations to help determine the precise overlaps and boundaries between the two conditions. Because children with Schizoid Personality Disorder are, in general, less handicapped, their symptoms are more subtle than those we typically observe in AS/HFA and therefore more difficult to diagnose. Parents or environmental factors are more likely to be blamed for Schizoid Personality Disorder because the organic nature of this disability is less clear. Many intervention approaches that are effective with AS/HFA can also be used with this group, but they require an understanding of the differences between these groups and a recognition that those with Schizoid Personality Disorders are often more socially skilled and independent, even thought they still require assistance and support in these areas.

Nonverbal Learning Disability (NLD)

Byron Rourke has popularized the concept of NLD (Rourke, 1989, 1995; Rourke & Tsatsanis, 2000). Based on his own research and earlier observations about individuals who have difficulty comprehending social information in their environments, he has proposed a model of right hemisphere dysfunction that results in a distinct neuropsychological profile and behavior.

According to Rourke, individuals with this disorder have intact auditory perception and rote verbal learning. Deficits include tactile perception (usually more marked on the left side of the body), visual perception, concept formation, and nonverbal problem-solving, particularly in novel situations. Intonation and inflection of speech and pragmatic language are additional difficulties. Academic deficits tend to be in mechanical arithmetic, mathematical reasoning, and reading comprehension, while abilities to decode and spell words are intact. Academic subject areas such as history or science can also be impaired because of reading comprehension and nonverbal problem-solving deficits. Other functional difficulties characterizing these individuals are poor social perception and judgment, which result in poor interaction skills. There can be a marked increase in social withdrawal and isolation as they grow older because of unsuccessful interpersonal experiences, and the group is at significant risk for depression and anxiety.

It can be seen that the social and pragmatic language deficits described in NLD are consistent with descriptions of AS. Klin et al. (1995) indicated that while many individuals with AS fit the profile of NLD, the reverse is not necessarily the case, since NLD is associated with a number of different conditions, both developmental and acquired (Rourke & Tsatsanis, 2000).

There are, however, differences between Rourke's description of NLD and the current understanding of AS. Rourke reports that children with NLD have noticeably delayed early language milestones (Rourke, 1995), while at least by current definition this is not true of individuals with AS (APA, 1994). Rourke describes significant visual-motor and visual-perceptual deficits as a defining feature of children with NLD, while Lincoln et al. (1998) and Manjivionia and Prior (1999) report that this is not a consistent, much less universal finding among subjects with AS. Also, Rourke describes "progressive deterioration" of "socialemotional adaptation" in NLD (1995, p. 24), while many authors who write about AS indicate that these factors improve over time (Fein et al., 1999; Lord & Ventner, 1992). Finally, Rourke indicates that NLD is associated with poor mechanical arithmetic skills, while the work of Minshew and colleagues (1997) indicates that these skills are generally well-developed in adults with HFA. (Since Minshew et al. did not study individuals diagnosed with AS, this may represent a distinguishing factor between HFA and AS/NLD, or it may represent a difference between AS/HFA and NLD.)

Overall, the concept of NLD may be a helpful model for analyzing the social and pragmatic difficulties associated with AS, but it does not appear to represent the same disorder.

Pervasive Developmental Disorder–Not Otherwise Specified (PDD-NOS)

In the DSM-IV, autism and AS are included in the category of Pervasive Developmental Disorder (PDD). This broad category also includes a "Not Otherwise Specified" diagnosis for situations in which there are prominent symptoms of autism or AS but full diagnostic criteria are not met, or when there is insufficient information to establish one of these more specific diagnoses.

Thus, a diagnosis of PDD-NOS can indicate that a person has some, but not all of the symptoms of autism or AS. Unfortunately, the diagnosis of PDD-NOS does not convey which symptoms are present and to what extent. Specifically, according to the DSM-IV, any one of the three categories of symptoms that characterize autism (that is, social deficits, communication deficits, and unusual behaviors/interests) can form the basis for a diagnosis of PDD-NOS. Ironically, this very broad definition is due to a minor wording change in the final draft of the DSM-IV (Volkmar, 1997). Rather than requiring social impairment "and" communication or behavioral abnormalities, the final version used the word "or." The effect of this is to enable a PDD-NOS diagnosis to be used quite loosely, including for persons with adequate social skills and interests, which is potentially very confusing for a disorder closely related to autism. This problem has been rectified in the "text revision" version of DSM-IV.

Further confusing the diagnostic picture, some clinicians have used the label of PDD-NOS instead of autism because it is seen as more palatable or more appropriate when children are very young. Other clinicians use PDD-NOS as synonymous with AS. Some clinicians even argue that PDD-NOS is the most appropriate diagnostic label for all impairments in reciprocal social interactions and the capacity to develop empathy, even among those who might otherwise be diagnosed with a conduct disorder or anti-social personality.

Although it is sometimes confusing, nonspecific, or misused, the PDD-NOS diagnostic category is, nevertheless, important because it enables clinicians to offer a diagnosis to those clients in need of services, but who do not fit neatly into the more specific categories that have been developed.

SUMMARY AND CONCLUSION

The DSM-IV diagnostic criteria for autism and AS overlap to a significant degree. The main differentiating features involve early developmental patterns, but for a variety of reasons this may not provide an adequate foundation for differential diagnosis. It is well-accepted that the characteristics of autism vary significantly in different individuals, ranging from extreme aloofness, lack of language, and limited nonverbal and adaptive skills (Wing, 2000) to awkward sociability, above-average intelligence and verbal fluency, and adequate vocational and community living skills. The terms HFA and AS are generally used to describe the upper end of this continuum, but professionals disagree whether these terms are interchangeable.

Psychological Assessment of Asperger Syndrome

Joel is an 8 year old who has been home-schooled since early in his Kindergarten year, when his parents withdrew him from the public school because he was being disciplined or sent home almost daily because of "behavior problems." He was described by the school as aggressive and hyperactive. This mystified his parents, who had never seen any difficult behaviors from him. At home, Joel was quiet and extremely polite. The family followed a quiet, orderly routine; it almost seemed as if the family consisted of three adults. Now that Joel was older, his family wanted to try a public school placement again. The school principal strongly recommended an evaluation before the school year began and offered to have the school system pay for it, so Joel's parents decided to have him seen by a psychologist who had helped their neighbor's son when he was having adjustment problems at the time of his parents' divorce.

DeMonte is a somewhat overweight 14-year-old boy who is finishing his freshman year of high school. He lives with his mother in a small, quiet, clean apartment. When the telephone rings, his mother knows it is for her, since she long ago realized that no one ever called for DeMonte. He has not been invited to a birthday party since very early childhood, he never talks about people in his classes at school, and he spends his evenings and weekends constructing model airplanes. If his mother would let him, he would talk to her about military aircraft for hours at a time. DeMonte did well in school when he was younger, but had increasing difficulty in middle school and is failing most of his high school classes. He has never received any special services at school – but just recently his mother had signed permission forms for him to be evaluated for the first time.

Rico is a 20-year-old student at a local university. Although he is managing his academic classes fairly well, he has had a series of roommates who soon ask to be transferred to different living situations. Rico's clothes and other personal possessions are piled all over the room, he never makes his bed, and he has been inconsistent about doing laundry, showering, and brushing his teeth. In contrast, his enormous collection of Car and Driver magazines is carefully organized, and after he looks at each issue he re-files it. He became very upset when his most recent roommate put an issue back in the wrong place, and caused such a scene that the dorm advisor took him to the Student Health Services walk-in clinic. There the psychologist on call raised the possibility of Asperger Syndrome for the first time and recommended an evaluation.

INTRODUCTION

As discussed in the previous chapter, there is disagreement among professionals about whether the diagnosis of AS should exist separate from HFA, and if so, what its defining features should be. Further, the question "does this person have AS/HFA?" is usually not the stated reason for referral to a general clinician; instead, individuals who might have AS/HFA are typically referred because of various behavioral or emotional symptoms, such as not following school or job site rules, having frequent tantrums, or not having any friends. How are psychologists to assess these individuals in order to be helpful to them and their families? Answering this question is the focus of this chapter.

Note that a medical evaluation by a physician knowledgeable about developmental disabilities is also an important part of establishing a diagnosis and treatment plan.

GOALS OF PSYCHOLOGICAL ASSESSMENT

Diagnosis

An assessment that leads to an appropriate diagnosis can be valuable for families. Diagnostic labels are sometimes criticized for detracting from clients' uniqueness and dignity. However, diagnoses can in fact serve multiple therapeutic functions.

First, they can help family members understand the individual better. Because persons with AS/HFA have average intelligence, it often happens that their actions are misinterpreted as intentional misbehavior. However, behaviors such as failing to follow directions, having tantrums, or acting in other socially unacceptable ways are usually a reflection of the person's AS/HFA. To know an individual has AS/HFA is to know that he or she has a neurologically-based disability, rather than deliberate misbehavior. Similarly, understanding the diagnosis can help parents stop blaming themselves as "bad" parents whose poor parenting skills have resulted in a misbehaving offspring. Further, parents can then help their other offspring deal with their feelings and concerns about their sibling's behavior. Finally, knowing and understanding the diagnosis allows parents to find ways to reduce the distress and maladaptive behaviors of the individual with AS/HFA, based on an understanding of the person's needs. For example, parents can learn that individuals with AS need help anticipating the sequence of events and activities that will occur, rather than being expected to cope with high degrees of spontaneity and unpredictability in family life. (See Chapter 4 for additional discussion of intervention strategies for AS/HFA.)

A second reason to assess for the purpose of diagnosis is to enable the individual to obtain services, such as special education, Vocational Rehabilitation, SSI, and other developmental disabilities supports. Almost without exception, a diagnosis and evaluation of current needs are required to determine eligibility for such programs. This sometimes creates a dilemma for parents. On one hand, they do not want their offspring to be unfairly stigmatized, so they sometimes resist disclosing diagnoses like AS/HFA. On the other hand, they generally recognize that their youngsters need help and understanding, which often is available only with one of the labels parents would rather avoid.

Diagnosis can also help families start to make plans for the future. Naturally, if the child is very young there are many decisions that cannot be made, but childhood is often not too early to give thought to issues such as the possible need for long-term supervision, guardianship, or financial supplements to income in adulthood.

Diagnostic labels can also help parents find other families with similar situations. For example, knowing only that a youngster has unusual interests, pedantic speech, and no friends does not enable parents to connect with parent support groups or advocacy organizations they can relate to. However, having a diagnosis of AS/HFA can more easily direct parents to other families with whom they have a lot in common, and who can provide tremendous emotional and practical support (such as listening to their feelings, supporting their perceptions, offering names of helpful dentists or barbers, summer camps, social skills groups, etc.). Related to this, knowing the diagnosis can also help parents find relevant resources such as books, websites, and support group meetings.

In summary, there are times when an assessment that concludes with an accurate diagnosis, emotional support, and recommendations of appropriate resources can be highly therapeutic and beneficial (Shea, 1984, 1993). A further goal for assessment, however, is to go beyond diagnosis to more detailed recommendations and intervention planning.

Intervention Planning

The assessment methods used to establish a diagnosis of AS/HFA understandably focus on the specific diagnostic criteria. Information about these factors alone, however, provides relatively little guidance for planning educational or other therapeutic interventions. Additional approaches are needed to answer questions about the unique ways in which AS is affecting the individual's ability to function successfully in school, work, community activities, etc. This information provides a foundation for developing individualized intervention plans (see Chapter 4).

PSYCHOLOGICAL ASSESSMENT PROCEDURES

Key parts of the assessment are obtaining from parents a developmental history and description of current behavior, interacting with the client directly, and formal testing. Since individuals with AS/HFA do not have mental retardation, it is particularly important for evaluations to go beyond intelligence testing and include additional measures that identify areas of impaired functioning.

Parent Interviews

Both for diagnostic purposes and intervention planning, parent interviews are vital. Further, it is extremely useful to have access to records that shed light on early development, such as notes from nursery school, report cards, and any previous testing.

For diagnostic purposes, it is important to obtain information about early language development. While we have seen that significant delays are not consistent with the DSM-IV criteria for AS, unusually mature-sounding, pedantic language, precocious reading skills, unusual vocal patterns and vocabulary use, and poor pragmatics are common (Baltaxe & Simmons, 1992). In terms of early social skills, there are generally difficulties in preschool, manifested in behavioral problems reflecting a lack of understanding of social norms and expectations, as well as sensory sensitivities and subtle difficulties processing and using language (Church et al., 2000). Early history for youngsters with AS/HFA will typically also reveal unusual interests and talents, such as memorizing television and movie dialogue, learning and talking a great deal about an obscure topic, or advanced musical or artistic skill.

The "gold standard" of structured parent interviews for obtaining information about past and current characteristics of autism is the Autism Diagnostic Interview–Revised (Lord et al., 1994). However, this instrument, originally developed for research purposes and still primarily used in that way, is not specific to AS/HFA and is probably too long and complex for general clinical use for this population.

Observation and Informal Interviews

Informal play or interviews will usually reveal some type of atypical behavior, such as:

- limited pretend play and social play by children
- poor joint attention (that is, following and using eye gaze to share interests with others)
- unusual social interactions (e.g., not responding to others, limited eye contact, poor conversational ability)
- disordered language (e.g., long monologues, unusual voice quality, loud speech)
- limited flexibility in changing tasks or topics
- unusual interests (in content and/or intensity)
- poor understanding of nonverbal cues to stop talking
- socially inappropriate behaviors (e.g., burping, passing gas) without apparent embarrassment
- unusual movements (e.g., flapping when excited)

Information from a child's teachers or other adult observers can also be useful and can often be gathered through a telephone interview. Particularly informative for diagnostic purposes is information about social skills, interests, and play skills in children:

- Does the individual have any friends?
- Does he or she seem interested in others but have difficulty approaching them and engaging them?
- Does the person want to talk about things others are not interested in?
- Does the individual do things that annoy others, and if so, does he or she seem to notice?
- For children: does the child play appropriately and use imagination in play?

For intervention planning, it is crucial also to gather information from both parents and teachers or other observers about the individual's unique strengths and difficulties:

- What skills are needed in order to become more independent in functioning in the community?
- What specific expectations is the individual not meeting? (such as sitting through circle time, obeying classroom rules, finishing work on time, turning in homework, accepting supervision and feedback)
- What special interests does the individual have that can be used to engage him/her in learning new skills?
- What modifications in academic expectations might be needed?
- What kinds of situations and stimulation create distress or agitation?
- What kinds of organizational strategies and structure have helped him/her be successful in meeting school or vocational expectations?

At times it may be useful to observe a child at school, if many behavior problems are occurring in that location. A school observation before the child meets the evaluator in the office or clinic is particularly useful, so that the child does not know he/she is the focus of the observation.

── **Formal Testing**

Psychological testing is a valuable part of the assessment process. It can supplement the clinician's judgment and perhaps counteract his/her biases and errors. It also provides specific information that cannot be obtained in other ways (such as standard scores that indicate how the individual's skills compare to those of others of the same age) and observations of how the person goes about completing tasks.

The most frequently used commercially available psychological tests used in studies of AS/HFA are discussed in the section that follows (see Appendix for publishers' contact information).

Cognitive Tests

Wechsler Scales

BACKGROUND

David Wechsler was a psychologist who devoted his career to the measurement of intelligence. Tests developed by him or built on the foundation of his work include the Wechsler Preschool and Primary Scale of Intelligence-Revised (WPPSI-R), the Wechsler Intelligence Scale for Children (now in its third edition, the WISC-III) and the Wechsler Adult Intelligence Scale (the current version is the WAIS-III). All of the Wechsler Scales consist of 10–14 subtests, divided between the "Verbal Scale" and the "Performance Scale." On the subtests that make up the Verbal scale, the examiner reads questions to the subject and writes down the subject's answers to be scored later. Verbal tasks include defining vocabulary words, repeating series of digits, and answering general information questions. The subtests on the Performance scale consist of a variety of tasks that use pictures, blocks, puzzles, or pencil and paper. Subjects do not need to speak to do these performance tasks, although they do need to understand the oral directions. The examiner reads directions to the subject and scores the work as correct or incorrect; on some tasks the subject's performance is timed because bonus points are given for speedy, correct work and subjects are penalized for working too slowly.

A score (called a "scaled score") comparing the subject's work to that of other people of the same age can be obtained for every subtest. The summary score for the Verbal subtests together is called the "Verbal IQ" (VIQ) and the summary score for the Performance subtests together is the "Performance (PIQ)." The summary score for the entire test is the "Full Scale IQ."

Much has been written about whether there is a characteristic "autistic" pattern of subtest scores on the Wechsler tests (see Lincoln et al., 1995, and Siegel et al., 1996, for reviews). Many studies have found that among people with autism, the highest Performance subtest is usually Block Design (using blocks to make geometric designs that match pictures), often with a high Object Assembly (non-interlocking puzzles) score too. The lowest Verbal subtest is generally Comprehension (answering questions involving knowledge and under-standing of social situations and institutions in our society); the lowest Performance score is generally Coding (a timed test involving copying marks according to a code at the top of the page). This profile, along with a VIQ markedly lower than PIQ, has been assumed by some to be a marker for the diagnosis of autism.

However, while this pattern is typical in populations of lower functioning individuals with autism, there is increasing evidence that among higher functioning individuals, the pattern of skills on Wechsler scales is more diverse than previously thought. Recent stud-ies have found all possible relationships between Verbal and Performance IQs: lower, higher, and equal. For example, Eaves et al. (1994) studied a group of 30 high functioning children with autism (mean VIQ = 72; mean PIQ = 74). Within this group, 43% had PIQ significantly higher than VIQ, but 32% had VIQ > PIQ, with 25% hav-ing VIQ not significantly different from PIQ.

Similarly, Siegel et al. (1996) reported results of a very rigorous study looking at individual profiles of subjects with high functioning autism and found much greater variability than previous reports sug-gested. Their sample consisted of 81 children and adults with care-fully diagnosed autism (individuals with no clear history of language delay, i.e. AS, were specifically excluded). Only subjects with Verbal, Performance, and Full Scale IQs > 70 were included. Instead of a uni-versal, typical pattern of VIQ < PIQ, this study found that 58% had VIQ > PIQ, 40% had PIQ > VIQ, and 2% (one child) had VIQ = PIQ. Similarly, among the adults, 64% had VIQ > PIQ while 36% had PIQ > VIQ. Statistically significant differences among children's VIQ vs. PIQ scores appeared in approximately the same number of cases in each direction, while significant differences among adults occurred more than twice as often in the direction of VIQ > PIQ. In terms of spe-cific subtests, fewer than 50% of either the children or adults had Block Design as their highest subtest or Comprehension as their lowest subtest.

Most of the studies looking at the question of a typical Wechsler profile were completed before AS was included as a diagnostic category in DSM-IV. So although it now seems clear that there is no definitive Wechsler profile of HFA, the question of whether there is a characteristic Wechsler profile in AS is not fully resolved (again, along with the broader question of whether AS is a distinct disorder from HFA).

Those who have described a typical AS profile suggest it includes a higher Verbal than Performance IQ, with strengths on Information and other language-related tasks, and weakness on timed visual-motor tasks, particularly Coding and Object Assembly (Ehlers et al., 1997; Klin et al., 2000). However, two recent studies of individuals carefully diagnosed according to DSM-IV criteria with either HFA or AS have found that the relationship of VIQ to PIQ was variable within both groups. Manjiviona and Prior (1999) found that the proportion of children with AS who had statistically significant differences between their Verbal and Performance IQ's was roughly the same as the proportion found in the typical population. When there were significant differences between the two IQ scores, VIQ > PIQ was the most common pattern in both the AS and HFA groups, although in both groups a substantial minority of children had the opposite pattern. While Ozonoff et al. (2000) reported that 50% of their subjects with AS had Verbal IQ's significantly higher than their Performance IQ's, 35% of those with HFA demonstrated this pattern also. In addition, in that study only 5 of the 23 children with HFA and 3 of the 12 with AS had Block Design as their highest subtest (Information was most frequently the highest in both groups).

In summary, while the Wechsler scales can provide a great deal of excellent, psychometrically sound information about the cognitive skills of individuals with AS/HFA, there is no distinctive pattern that confirms or contradicts the diagnoses.

Stanford–Binet

BACKGROUND

Various forms of the Binet test have been used by psychologists since Alfred Binet's original work in the late 19th–early 20th century. The most recent version (1986) is the Stanford–Binet 4th edition; for the 26 years prior to its publication, the

Stanford–Binet, Form L-M was used. The L-M version and its
predecessors were organized by age level, and used different
tasks at each level. The resulting score was a "mental age"
equivalent that could be converted to an IQ. The 4th edition is
organized differently, using sets of test tasks in several areas
(Verbal Reasoning, Abstract/Visual Reasoning, Quantitative
Reasoning, and Short-Term Memory) that increase in difficulty,
just like the Wechsler subtests. The 4th edition of the
Stanford–Binet yields standard scores in each of the areas, and an
overall "Composite Score."

The 4th edition of the Stanford-Binet was used in a large study of
preschool children with one of four disorders: high or low functioning
autism, mental retardation without autism, or developmental language
disorders (Rapin, 1996). (Since the study focused on young children
with significant communication handicaps, it did not include children
who might be diagnosed with AS.) The high functioning group's mean
Abstract/Visual Reasoning subtest and area scores were in the average
range, while their mean Verbal Reasoning subtest and area scores were
$1-1\frac{1}{2}$ standard deviations below average. Thus, the Stanford–Binet 4th
edition in this study yielded the equivalent of the so-called characteristic Wechsler autism pattern (that is, VIQ < PIQ) in the HFA group. The
low-functioning autistic group, on the other hand, was equally delayed
in Abstract/Visual Reasoning and Verbal Reasoning. The authors
pointed out that the psychometric properties of the Stanford–Binet 4th
edition at this age level require cautious interpretation of results,
because scores can actually be higher for children who are unable to
perform certain tasks than for children who perform all tasks but make
some errors.

Harris et al. (1990) reported finding a characteristic profile of
subtest scores on the Stanford–Binet 4th edition, consisting of highest
scores on Pattern Analysis and lowest score on Absurdities, in both
high and low functioning young children (35–84 months) with autism.

Rapin and colleagues (1996) reported that on the Verbal
Absurdities subtest from the Stanford–Binet 4th edition in their study
of young children, the scores of children with HFA were significantly

lower than those of children with developmental language disorder matched in nonverbal intelligence.

Interestingly, several subtests from the Stanford–Binet L-M edition were shown in a study by Rumsey and Hamburger (1990) to have excellent ability to discriminate ten men with HFA from two different control groups. The subtests were Verbal Absurdities, Picture Absurdities, Problem Situations, and Plan of Search, which occur between the VII–XIII year levels. Groups of normal controls and adults with dyslexia achieved between 90 and 100% correct responses, while the subjects with HFA scored significantly lower, with the mean scores on all subtests except Picture Absurdities being below 50%. Similarly, Form L-M Picture Absurdities and Verbal Absurdities were reported by Minshew et al. (1997) to discriminate adults with HFA from normal controls. Manjiviona and Prior (1999) reported that in their sample of children (ages 6–17 years) with HFA or AS, many had significant difficulty with the Form L-M Verbal Absurdities and Problem Situations; mean percentage correct ranged from 40 to 71%. The subtests did not differentiate the two clinical groups from each other, except for a trend for children diagnosed with autism to score more poorly on Problem Situations than those diagnosed with AS.

Kaufman Assessment Battery for Children (K-ABC)

BACKGROUND

The K-ABC was published in 1983 by Alan and Nadeen Kaufman. Dr. Alan Kaufman is a leading expert and scholar in the area of psychological testing who has done extensive writing and research on the Wechsler scales.

The K-ABC is based on a theory of intelligence and cognition that is different from the Wechsler model of Verbal and Performance. According to Kaufman and others, there are two basic information processing styles: Simultaneous processing, which is thought to be reflected on nonverbal, visual-spatial tasks, and tasks that involve taking in many elements of information at the same time, and Sequential processing, which is reflected in verbal, analytic, step-by-step information processing.

A few studies were published between 1985 and 1991 looking at whether this measure of Simultaneous vs. Sequential skills sheds light on the nature of cognitive skills and deficits in children with autism spectrum disorders. The results of the various studies were inconsistent, and no recent studies of AS/HFA have used this measure. The K-ABC is still used clinically, mainly as a measure of nonverbal intelligence, since a number of its subtests do not require expressive language from the child.

Freeman et al. (1985) looked at performance on the K-ABC in a study of children with autism who had a mean VIQ of 90 on the WISC-R. In their sample there was no significant difference between the group means on K-ABC Simultaneous vs. Sequential processing scores. Where individual differences were found, the Sequential scores were higher than Simultaneous scores, contrary to the hypothesis that autism is associated with relatively poor sequential, analytic, "left-brain" skills.

Allen et al. (1991) also studied a group of HFA children with the K-ABC and WISC-R. In their study all the HFA children were found to have PIQ > VIQ (means of 84.6 and 56.7, respectively) and most had Simultaneous processing scores greater than Sequential processing scores (means of 89.5 and 75.1 respectively), consistent with the authors' hypothesis. The authors speculated that the Sequential vs. Simultaneous difference on the K-ABC was not found in the Freeman et al. (1985) study because of differences between the two samples of subjects studied. Subjects in the Freeman et al. study had higher Verbal IQ's, which are correlated with higher Sequential processing scores. Thus, Allen et al. suggested, for those subjects Sequential scores were equal to or higher than Simultaneous scores, but in a more typical, verbally-handicapped group, relative Simultaneous strengths were seen.

The Allen et al. (1991) study also analyzed the subjects' performance according to a previously formulated (Naglieri et al., 1983) concept of "WISC-R Processing Scales" (WISC-R-P). The WISC-R subtests of Picture Completion, Block Design, and Object Assembly were proposed to constitute Simultaneous subtests, with Digit Span and Coding reflecting Sequential processing. A correlational analysis supported this clustering of WISC-R subtests. The authors concluded that "the study demonstrated the utility of the K-ABC and the WISC-R Simultaneous processing scales in assessing the nonverbal cognitive potentials of these language-impaired children" (p. 499).

Academic Achievement

Any of the standard achievement tests (e.g., Woodcock-Johnson III Tests of Achievement, Wechsler Individual Achievement Test, Second Edition, Kaufman Test of Educational Achievement) can be used to assess the academic skill levels of students with AS/HFA. The most important point for psychologists to make clear is that skills are likely to be quite scattered, so that they are not well-represented by summary scores.

A number of studies (see Goldstein et al., 1994; Minshew et al., 1994; Minshew et al., 1997) have indicated that certain mechanical or procedural skills, such as attention, simple memory, simple language, and spelling are relatively well-preserved or even above average in students with AS/HFA, while more complex skills such as reading comprehension, complex memory and reasoning, applying computation skills to mathematical problems, and writing reports and stories are relatively weaker. Most achievement tests look at both kinds of skills then combine scores on related tasks into summary scores, which may not reflect either the child's significant strengths or marked weaknesses. A good example of this is in reading, where children with AS/HFA generally do very well with word attack (decoding) skills, but poorly with comprehension. It is important that clinicians recognize this and look carefully at individual skills reflected on various test tasks, rather than relying on summary scores.

Extensive information about academic testing and remediation for students with AS can be found in Myles and Simpson (1998) and in Siegel et al. (1996). See also Chapter 4 for additional intervention resources.

Adaptive Behavior

BACKGROUND

The term "adaptive behavior" refers to skills that a person actually uses, independently and on a regular basis, to meet the expectations of daily life in his/her community. It has long been recognized that the kinds of skills measured by intelligence, academic, and language tests do not necessarily translate into daily independent functioning. In some cases, individuals may have limited intellectual and academic skills, but be very competent in managing their daily lives. Alternatively, some individuals have a large store of knowledge and other abilities that lead to high test scores, but have difficulty meeting the challenges and demands of daily self-care and community life.

The most commonly used adaptive behavior measure is the Vineland Adaptive Behavior Scales. (Others include the Adaptive Behavior Assessment System and the Scales of Independent Behavior-Revised.)

The Vineland and other adaptive behavior tests are typically scored based on a semi-structured interview with the individual's parents or other caregivers. (Often an alternate form is available for teachers.) On the Vineland, scores are obtained in the areas of Communication, Daily Living Skills, and Socialization, as well as an overall summary score called the "Adaptive Behavior Composite." There is also a listing of maladaptive behaviors that can be evaluated, and for young children, items involving fine and gross motor skills.

An assessment of adaptive skills is a very important part of the assessment of AS/HFA because adaptive behavior is often the area in which the handicaps associated with AS/HFA are most obvious. It is not unusual clinically to see adults with IQs in the average or even superior range, (that is, 100 or higher) but adaptive behavior scores in the 60's, 50's, or even 40's. Problems related to AS/HFA, such as limited social skills and interests, poor organizational skills that affect daily hygiene and self-care, unusual sensory interests and aversions, and pragmatic communication deficits are often (but not always) tapped by adaptive behavior measures.

The typical pattern of Vineland domain scores seen in individuals with autism involves a significant deficit in Socialization and relative strengths in Daily Living Skills, with Communication scores falling somewhere in between (Carter et al., 1998). According to these authors, this pattern of scatter may be less pronounced in autistic individuals with average IQs (that is, AS/HFA), but problems in Socialization and a large number of maladaptive behaviors are typical.

Szatmari et al. (1995) used the Vineland as part of a battery of tests with a sample of preschool children with AS or autism, all with nonverbal intelligence above the range of mental retardation. Although the mean Leiter (nonverbal) IQ of the children with AS was 99, their mean Vineland scores ranged from 71 (Activities of Daily Living) to 83 (Communication). The Vineland scores of the autism group were significantly lower than those of the children diagnosed with AS except in the Motor domain in which the two groups were equivalent.

Similarly, Rapin (1996) reported that while the average nonverbal IQ of the young children with HFA in their study was 103, their Vineland scores ranged from around 70 (Activities of Daily Living and Socialization) to around 80 (Communication and Motor).

Checklists and Rating Scales

The *Asperger Syndrome Diagnostic Scale* (ASDS) (Myles & Simpson, 1998) is a new instrument for children ages 5–18 that yields an "AS Quotient" reflecting the likelihood that the youngster has AS. It is a 50-item scale that can be completed by anyone who knows the child well, defined as having regular sustained contact for at least two weeks. The scale was normed on 227 individuals with disorders that include AS, autism, AD/HD, learning disabilities, and behavior disorders.

Autism Spectrum Screening Questionnaire (ASSQ). This is a 27-item checklist designed to be completed by parents or teachers to screen youngsters age 6–17 years for AS. It appears to be a very useful tool for obtaining information that can assist in diagnosis. Because it is new, there is only a small amount of research using it, but the authors (Ehlers et al., 1999) found that it could differentiate youngsters with clinically diagnosed AS from those with disruptive behavior disorders or learning disabilities. They described use of the ASSQ in a sample of 110 consecutive referrals to a neuropsychiatric clinic. The authors' recommended cutoff score for parent ratings identified

62% of youngsters clinically diagnosed with AS, with a 10% false positive rate. The recommended cutoff score for teacher ratings identified 70% of subjects with AS, with a 9% false positive rate.

Australian Scale for Asperger Syndrome (ASAS). This scale, developed by Tony Attwood, is a non-normed instrument of 24 items to be rated by frequency of occurrence, plus 10 additional items scored as present/absent. It is intended for use with children in "primary school years." There are no specific cut-off scores, but the author suggests that if a majority of items are indicated as occurring more than "rarely," the child should be seen for further evaluation.

Autism Screening Questionnaire (ASQ). This is a 40-item screening questionnaire adapted from items from the best available diagnostic interview measure, the Autism Diagnostic Interview-Revised (ADI; Lord et al., 1994). The ASQ has been shown to have good ability to discriminate autism spectrum disorders from non-spectrum disorders. It appears to have good potential for use with individuals with AS/HFA as well as with lower-functioning individuals who may not have autism. In a study of 200 individuals with a variety of neuropsychiatric diagnoses, the recommended cutoff identified 85% of individuals diagnosed with autism spectrum disorders, with a false positive rate of 25% (Berument et al., 1999). Like the other questionnaires reviewed in this section, it is designed for screening only, not for diagnosis.

Tests of Executive Function

"Executive Function" is a term that has been used to refer to the range of cognitive abilities that are similar to the work of a business executive: planning, organizing, monitoring progress, staying focused, controlling impulses, shifting strategies as needed, and evaluating outcomes. Deficits in Executive Function have been identified in a number of clinical populations, including those with Attention Deficit/ Hyperactivity Disorder, Tourette syndrome, and frontal lobe lesions (Benetto et al., 1996; Ozonoff, 1998). There has been increasing interest in recent years about the relationship of Executive Function deficits to

AS/HFA; several test instruments have been the focus of most of the research.

Wisconsin Card Sort Test

BACKGROUND

> The Wisconsin Card Sort Test (WCST) consists of 128 cards containing simple symbols that vary along the dimensions of color, number, and shape (for example, two blue squares, three red triangles). Subjects are asked to match the cards, one at a time, to one of four sample cards. The examiner gives the subject feedback after each card is placed, indicating whether it is correct or incorrect, but during the course of the test the correct matching strategy changes without notice to the subject (for example, at first cards should be matched by color, but at some point they should be matched by shape). Various aspects of the subject's performance are scored, including number of categories completed, errors based on failing to continue using correct categories, and errors based on perseverating on a previous categorization strategy after it is no longer correct. The test is generally considered to be a measure of cognitive flexibility.

There is substantial evidence that individuals with AS/HFA have difficulty with the aspects of executive functioning tapped by this instrument, which can be important information for documentation of impaired functioning and/or intervention planning. However, the WCST is less useful for diagnostic purposes, because research to date has not identified a cutoff score or level of skill on this task specific to AS/HFA.

A number of studies of AS/HFA have included the WCST in the battery of neuropsychological tests. The most common findings are that subjects with AS/HFA perseverate more (Benetto et al., 1996; Ozonoff, 1995, Ozonoff & Jensen, 1999; Ozonoff et al., 1991; Szatmari et al., 1989) or complete fewer categories (Rumsey, 1985; Rumsey & Hamburger 1988, 1990) than control subjects, although these findings are not universal (e.g., Minshew et al., 1992, 1997). Many of the research studies do not make reference to the norms of the test, and in fact one study (Ozonoff, et al. 1991) found the degree of perseveration of subjects with HFA to be within normal limits according to test norms, even though statistically it was significantly higher than the performance of the clinical control group.

A very interesting study (Berger et al., 1993), looking at young Dutch adults with autism spectrum disorders and normal or near-normal IQs, found that out of a variety of cognitive measures, performance on a Dutch card-sorting task analogous to the WCST was the best predictor of progress in social understanding (as measured by a task of interpreting pictures of social situations).

The WCST is now available in a computerized version, which eliminates the administration and scoring difficulties examiners might experience. However, a study by Ozonoff (1995) indicated that the computerized and standard administration versions are not equivalent for HFA children, who performed much better on the computerized version. There is also a new, shorter (64 card) version of the WCST.

Rey–Osterrieth Complex Figure Test

BACKGROUND

This simple test requires the subject to copy, then later recall and reproduce a complicated geometric design. The copying task is considered to be a measure of organizational abilities, while the delayed recall task also includes a memory component.

Studies have found no significant difference between subjects with AS/HFA and controls on the copying component (Manjiviona and Prior, 1999; Minshew et al., 1992, 1997; Rumsey & Hamburger, 1990) but there is some indication that subjects with HFA perform significantly less well than controls on the delayed recall task. This finding is consistent with results on various other types of tasks in suggesting that on some simple information processing tasks people with autism spectrum disorders do not differ from controls, but they demonstrate significantly deficient performance on more complex information processing tasks.

Tower of Hanoi/Tower of London

BACKGROUND

> These measures use the same essential materials (three rings or
> beads graded in size from small to large, and three pegs) and task
> (moving the rings/beads from the starting peg to a goal peg, in as
> few moves as possible, without ever placing a larger object on top
> of a smaller one). Successful completion of the task requires
> substantial planning ability.

Several studies (Bennetto et al., 1995; Berthier, 1995; Ozonoff &
Jensen, 1999; Ozonoff et al., 1991) have reported significantly less
efficient performance by subjects with AS/HFA compared to clinical
or normal controls.

Trail Making

BACKGROUND

> This timed paper and pencil test is part of the Halstead-Reitan
> Neuropsychological Battery. Trail Making A is essentially a
> "connect the dots" task, in which the subject is asked to connect
> randomly scattered numbers in correct sequence. Trail Making B
> involves connecting both numbers and letters (for example,
> 1-A-2-B-3-C etc.) and is considered to be a measure of reasoning
> and cognitive flexibility.

Research to date indicates that, as with other Executive Function
tests, the Trail Making Test does not contribute significantly to making
the diagnosis of AS, but may be useful in documenting organiza-
tional/planning difficulties in a particular individual.

Rumsey and Hamburger (1988) found that adult men with
AS/HFA were significantly slower than controls on both A and B,

although the difference might have been partly due to slightly different IQs in the two groups. Minshew et al. (1997) also found that subjects with HFA performed worse (i.e. slower) than controls on Trail Making A, consistent with inefficient psychomotor skills. The difference between subjects with HFA and controls on Trail Making B, while observable, did not reach statistical significance, but this may have been due to unusual psychometric characteristics in the control group.

Other Measures

Nepsy. A new instrument on the market that appears to have good potential for measuring the neuropsychological status of children ages 3–12 years is the NEPSY (short for Neuropsychology). This test is composed of a large number of subtests that can be used in various combinations as measures of Attention/Executive Function, Language, Sensorimotor Functions, Visuospatial Processing, and Memory and Learning. A significant advantage of the NEPSY is that it is a complete package of standardized materials (including a version of the Tower of Hanoi/London), directions, and norms for children.

The NEPSY manual contains a brief description of a study of 23 children described as having "autistic-type disorders" and IQs over 80. Results included overall deficits compared to controls on some aspects of Attention/Executive Function (specifically, marked difficulties with planning, cognitive flexibility, and productivity, but adequate visual and auditory attention, impulse control, and motor persistence) and Memory (difficulty with memory for faces, narrative memory, and list learning), as well as certain specific subtests in other domains.

Autism Diagnostic Observation Schedule – (ADOS). This instrument, developed by Lord et al. (2000) is the counterpart of the "gold standard" ADI-R. It is a standardized set of materials and situations designed to elicit social and communication behaviors and skills to aid in the diagnosis of autism. Originally designed for research purposes and available only after extensive training from the authors, it is now commercially available for general clinical use (see Appendix) although it is quite expensive as well as being complex to learn. There is not a specific algorithm (that is, formula and cut-off score) for a diagnosis of AS, as there is for autism.

Child Behavior Checklist. In addition to the test instruments discussed in this chapter, a broad measure of emotional/behavioral disorders such as the Child Behavior Checklist (Achenbach, 1991; Achenbach & Rescorla, 2000) can be useful in screening for additional disorders that also require intervention.

Stroop Color Word Test

BACKGROUND

In the Stroop Color Word Test subjects are asked to read a list of color names that are printed in a different color (e.g., the word GREEN is printed in blue).

Although this test has been shown to be sensitive to some clinical conditions (such as Attention Deficit/Hyperactivity Disorder; Ozonoff & Jensen, 1999), it has never been found to differentiate persons with AS/HFA from controls.

Tests under Development

Ghuman-Folstein Screen for Social Interaction. This recently developed rating scale of social behaviors in preschool children (Ghuman et al., 1998) also shows promise as a screening tool. It has been found by its authors to be capable of differentiating children with autism spectrum disorders from typically developing children and from children with other developmental disabilities. However, the authors cautioned that this instrument is still under development and does not yet have the research foundation to be used clinically as a screening tool.

The Ghuman et al. study involved 60 normally developing controls and 51 children with various developmental disorders, some of whom met criteria for autism on one or more elements of the ADI-R.

The rating scale was able to differentiate control children from the clinical group. More importantly for the purpose of differentiating AS/HFA from other developmental disorders, within the clinical group the mean screening instrument scores of children who met criteria on the ADI-R were significantly lower than those of children who did not. However, the absolute difference in scores was very small, the sample size of this study was small, and the clinical group was heterogeneous, leading to the authors' conclusion that more research is needed to validate the use of the test for clinical purposes.

DISCO. The DISCO (Diagnostic Interview for Social and Communication Disorders) is being developed by Lorna Wing and Judith Gould as a semi-structured interview for collecting information about development and behavior from birth. It is relevant for all autism spectrum disorders and other related developmental disorders, and is designed both to provide diagnostic information and to identify intervention needs.

Gilliam Asperger's Disorder Scale. This instrument will be published in 2001.

Tests in Other Areas

Language Tests. For both diagnostic and intervention purposes, standard measures of expressive and receptive language (e.g., PLS-3, CELF-3, TACL, Rossetti, Communication and Symbolic Behavior Scales, Test of Language Competence-Extended Version) and a sample of spontaneous communication are appropriate components of an initial evaluation of a young child suspected of an autism spectrum disorder.

Resources for information about assessment of language functions in AS include Filipek et al. (1999) and Marans (1997).

Measure of Motor Skills. While there is no good evidence that motor skills differentiate AS from HFA (Ozonoff and Griffith, 2000), motor testing by an occupational therapist and/or physical therapist may be very important for intervention planning purposes. Many youngsters with AS/HFA need modified expectations (such as reduced requirements for handwriting) and/or additional instruction or support for learning motor-based skills (such as handwriting practice, typing instruction, Adaptive Physical Education).

SUMMARY OF RECOMMENDATIONS FOR ASSESSMENT

In the assessment of AS, as in other psychological assessments, the specific battery of tests to be administered should be selected based on the referral question and any related issues that the psychologist anticipates. For example, is the family asking about diagnosis, intervention recommendations, or both?

Generally, it should be anticipated that at a minimum the psychological assessment of suspected AS/HFA will consist of:

- parent interview, adaptive assessment, and for youngsters, parental rating scale information (CBCL and an Asperger/autism scale)
- teacher information in some form (rating scales, telephone interview, school observation, letter, or informal questionnaire)
- intelligence testing if, as is generally the case, there is an indication of problems with school or vocational performance, or if required by service agencies
- academic achievement testing under the same circumstances as intellectual assessment
- a test of language comprehension if there is any indication of "non-compliance" or school performance difficulties (note: this might be more appropriately performed by a speech/language therapist, along with an assessment of expressive and pragmatic language skills)

Additional testing that may be helpful if there are questions about intervention needs and eligibility:

- a test of motor skills (may indicate the need for Adaptive Physical Education, occupational therapy, modified vocational plans, etc.)

- Executive Function neuropsychological tests (WCST, Tower of London/Hanoi) that may help demonstrate or explain the student's difficulty with cognitive flexibility or planning/organizing

AFTER THE ASSESSMENT

No assessment is complete until the questions that prompted the assessment have been answered. An important part of answering parents' questions is the interpretive session in which staff and parents sit down together to discuss the findings, recommendations, and feelings generated by the assessment (Shea, 1984, 1993). In addition, professionals involved in the assessment should play a major role in explaining evaluation results and advocating for services with schools, agencies, and other service providers who may be unfamiliar with AS/HFA (Volkmar & Klin, 2000).

SUMMARY AND CONCLUSIONS

Evaluation of AS/HFA by a psychologist, in collaboration with professionals from other disciplines (generally speech/language, occupational therapy, and medicine) provides a foundation for educational and therapeutic interventions for individuals with AS/HFA and their families. Establishing the diagnosis, identifying strengths and needs, and interpreting these to families, teachers, and other service providers are key elements of the assessment process. Evaluations should include information from parents and teachers/caregivers, observation and interaction with the client, and formal testing with specific instruments selected based on the questions and goals of the assessment.

APPENDIX

Some tests are available from more than one publisher; the least expensive sources we could find, based on 2001 catalogue prices, are listed here.

Cognitive Tests

The Wechsler scales are available from Psychological Corporation, 800 211-8378 or http://www.psychcorp.com. Approximate prices: WPPSI-R $665; WISC-III $675; WAIS-III $700.

The Stanford–Binet 4th edition and some Stanford-Binet L-M materials are available from Riverside Publishing Company, 800 323-9540 or http://www.riverpub.com. The approximate price of the 4th edition is $744. For the three most discriminating subtests of the L-M edition (Verbal Absurdities, Problem Situations, and Plan of Search), the materials needed are Record Form (approximate price $57) and Manual for the Third Edition (approximate price $70). The only available source for Picture Absurdities is the Stanford–Binet 4th edition; materials needed are Guide for Administering and Scoring (approximate price $69.50), Item 3 Book (approximate price $127) and record booklets (approximate price $78.50).

The K-ABC is available from American Guidance Service, 800 328-2560 or http://www.agsnet.com. Approximate price $393.

Academic Achievement Tests

The Woodcock–Johnson III Tests of Achievement is available from Riverside Publishing Company, 800 323-9540 or http://www.riverpub.com. Approximate price $425.

The Wechsler Individual Achievement Test, Second Edition, is available from The Psychological Corporation, 800 211-8378 or http://www.psychcorp.com. Approximate price $300.

The Kaufman Test of Educational Achievement NU (Normative Update) is available from American Guidance Service 800 328-2560 or http://www.agsnet.com. Approximate price $265.

Adaptive Behavior Tests

The Vineland Adaptive Behavior Scales are available from American Guidance Service, 800 328-2560 or http://www.agsnet.com. Approximate prices $85 for the parent interview survey form; $55 for the classroom edition. Supplemental norms for individuals with autism were published in the Journal of Autism and Developmental Disorders, 1998, 28, 287–302.

The Adaptive Behavior Assessment System is available from The Psychological Corporation, 800 211–8378 or http://www.psychcorp.com. Approximate price $139 for the School Kit, $99 for the Adult version.

The Scales of Independent Behavior-Revised is available from Riverside Publishing Company, 800 323-9540 or http://www. riverpub.com. Approximate price is $193.

Checklists and Rating Scales

The ASDS is available from Pro-Ed, 800 897-3202 or http://www.proedinc.com. Approximate price: $89.

The ASSQ by Ehlers, Gillberg, and Wing was published in the Journal of Autism and Developmental Disorders, 1999, 29, 129–141.

The ASAS is included in Asperger's Syndrome: A Guide for Parents and Professionals by Tony Attwood (1994; Jessica Kingsley Publishers).

The ASQ is described in the British Journal of Psychiatry, 1999, 444–451, and will soon be published by Western Psychological Services, 800 648-8857 or http://www.wpspublish.com.

Tests of Executive Function

The Wisconsin Card Sort Test is available from Psychological Assessment Resources, 800 331-TEST (8378) or http://www.parinc.com. Approximate prices: $250 for standard version; $639 for the 128 card computerized version, $475 for the 64 card computerized version.

The Rey-Osterrieth Complex Figure Test and Recognition Trial is available from Psychological Assessment Resources, 800 331-TEST (8378) or http://www.parinc.com. Approximate price is $195.

The Tower of Hanoi is not commercially available (except in the NEPSY), although a description of the materials is contained in a published article (Borys et al., 1982). A computerized version is available from Western Psychological Services, 800 648-8857 or http://www.wpspublish.com, but there is no published information about the equivalence of this administration method for individuals with AS/HFA. Materials for the Tower of London are available from MHS, 800 456-3003 or http://www.mhs.com. Approximate price $205.

The Trail Making Test (versions for adults and for children ages 9–14 years) is available from Reitan Neuropsychology Laboratory, 800 882-2022 or email reitanlab@aol.com. Approximate price: $50.

Other Tests

NEPSY: A Developmental Neuropsychological Assessment is available from the Psychological Corporation, 800 211-8378 or http://www.psychcorp.com. Approximate price $561.

The ADOS-G is available from Western Psychological Services, 800 648-8857 or http://www.wpspublish.com. Approximate price: $1325.

The Child Behavior Checklists and related materials are now available as the Achenbach System of Empirically Based Assessment from the University of Vermont, 802 656-8313 or http://ASEBA.UVM.edu.

The Ghuman–Folstein Screen for Social Interaction is not yet commercially available. Contact Jaswinder Kaur Ghuman, M.D., Department of Psychiatry, The Kennedy Krieger Institute, The John Hopkins University, School of Medicine, 1750 E. Fairmount Avenue, Baltimore, MD 21231 for more information.

DISCO (Diagnostic Interview for Social and Communication Disorders) is not yet commercially available. The contact for information from Dr. Lorna Wing's group is Carole Murray, Elliot House, 113 Masons Hill, Bromley, Kent BR2 9HT, England. Email Cmurray@nas.org.uk.

The Gilliam Asperger's Disorder Scale will be published in 2001 by Pro-Ed, 800 897-3202 or http://www.proedinc.com.

4

Interventions

The recent, substantial increase in the number of people with AS/HFA has mobilized parents, school personnel, and other professionals to develop a range of intervention approaches to meet these individuals' needs. However, the research literature on this topic is sparse, so interventions generally lack a solid empirical base. Nevertheless, clinicians must still address the pressing needs for adaptations and interventions. This chapter will describe principles and strategies of interventions that have grown out of clinical needs and been found by teachers, psychologists, parents, and others to be widely helpful. We will also review applied research studies and discuss the implications of research for clinical practice. Resources for additional and updated information are also included.

Research studies have consistently emphasized the link between structured environments and positive outcomes for students with autism spectrum disorders (Rutter & Bartak, 1973; Mesibov et al., 1994). For the purposes of this discussion, structure is defined as direction by teacher, parent, or other caregiver of where to be, what to do, how and how long to do it, and what to do next. These elements of structure have been a foundation of the TEACCH program's approach to autism spectrum disorders, including AS/HFA, for over 30 years. In fact, TEACCH's intervention techniques are called "Structured Teaching" (Kunce & Mesibov, 1998; Mesibov, 1994).

THEORETICAL FOUNDATIONS OF THE TEACCH STRUCTURED TEACHING METHOD FOR AUTISM SPECTRUM DISORDERS ━━━━━

Structured teaching interventions are based on the integration of two key sets of information: (1) an understanding of the neurologically-based patterns of thinking characteristic of autism in general; and (2) sensitive observation of the individual's skills, special interests, and areas of confusion or distress.

Understanding Autism Spectrum Disorders ━━━━━━━━━━━━━

The first important element for effective interventions is understanding autism, including AS/HFA. Although most parents and professionals involved with individuals on the autism spectrum readily acknowledge the neurological basis of the disorder, fewer examine the implications of a neurological disability for thinking, learning, and understanding. However, making the connection between the neurological impairments and functional difficulties is central to designing effective interventions.

The neurologically-based manifestations of AS/HFA, like those of lower functioning autism, involve difficulties in the areas of communication, social interactions, and atypical behavior and interests. As described in Chapter 2, communication difficulties are most noticeable in the form of poor pragmatic and social language, which compound academic and social difficulties. In addition to these expressive and nonverbal difficulties, clinical descriptions (Grandin, 1995) and research studies (Boucher & Lewis, 1989; Minshew et al., 1995) clearly describe the receptive language difficulties that some individuals with AS/HFA have, and how these can result in problems benefiting from verbal instruction and participating in social interactions.

Socially, although the person with AS/HFA might be interested in having friends and participating in social interactions, friendships are hard to form when social convention does not come easily, empathy is difficult to express, and emotional cues are hard to recognize. It is almost impossible for individuals with AS/HFA to keep up with the subtle social cues and rapidly changing activities and stimuli that characterize social interactions. Further, cues and reinforcements from aregivers can be difficult to identify and track, so typical praise and reward systems are often ineffective with these individuals.

Atypical interests and repetitive behaviors can also make group settings difficult for individuals with AS/HFA. The individual's interests are often unusual in their subject and intensity, so that others of the same age with more typical recreational interests might feel they have little in common. Behaviors such as pacing, finger rubbing, or making unusual noises often lead to rejection by peers. Also, the person with AS/HFA can become easily anxious or disorganized in overstimulating or unstructured situations, leading to outbursts or temper tantrums that may be difficult for parents, teachers, co-workers, or peers to understand. Related to this, changes in routine, welcomed by most others who enjoy a day off or a surprise outing, can be a source of stress and trigger inappropriate behavior, which further distances the individual with AS/HFA from his peers.

The unusual behaviors of persons with autism spectrum disorders must be understood to reflect neurological differences. Observers who view these behaviors as willful, stubborn, unmotivated, or oppositional are missing an essential point that must be understood in order for remediation to be effective: neurologically-based cognitive differences frequently result in behavioral problems.

Finally, there are cognitive difficulties frequently found with students that can make their school experience depressing and unproductive. For example, students with AS/HFA have shown deficits in abstractions (Minshew et al., 1995), sequential processing (Allen et al., 1991), holding information in working memory while considering other information (Bennetto et al., 1995), and integrating information from multiple sensory modalities (Rosenblatt et al., 1995). Further, organizing themselves in time, space, and behavior to meet school expectations can be very challenging.

Individual Observation and Planning

A second important component of a Structured Teaching approach is individualized assessment. A paradox of AS/HFA is that while experienced professionals can easily recognize the characteristics of AS/HFA, there is enormous variability among these individuals. So while the characteristics of AS/HFA described above are important for all parents and professionals to understand, it is also crucial that each person's pattern of understanding and ability be considered, in order to design effective interventions. Among individuals with AS/HFA, the wide variability in cognitive, social, and temperamental traits results in a range of behavioral styles, including shy and quiet personalities, intrusiveness, rigidity, disorganization, and every possible combination of these. Further, intellectual functioning can range from slightly below normal to gifted and talented.

Understanding the unique characteristics of these talented, though quite handicapped, individuals is essential. Combinations of formal normed assessments and informal observations of skills and strategies are necessary to get a complete picture of current functioning levels (see Chapter 3). This understanding can increase our tolerance of inappropriate behaviors and lead to more realistic expectations. It can also help us to develop more effective intervention strategies.

IMPLICATIONS OF AS/HFA FOR DESIGNING INTERVENTIONS ⎯⎯

1. As discussed previously, a person with AS/HFA has difficulty with one or more aspects of understanding and using language and related aspects of communication. This is inevitably true, even if the person talks a great deal and uses sophisticated vocabulary. Often auditory processing abilities are also affected, so that the individual has difficulty understanding complicated verbal directions or explanations. This problem is made worse when the person is already confused, upset, or overwhelmed by other stimulation. For example, in the following situations verbal explanations may be ineffective and may add to distress and behavior problems:

- explaining to a child why he cannot make his art project the way he wants to
- telling a student why he must wait 10 additional minutes in a hot costume before it is his turn to perform on stage

■   announcing to a work group that an uncompleted work project has been abruptly postponed and another one substituted

Another communication problem commonly seen in people with AS/HFA is that they understand language concretely. That is, words have one meaning only. This makes it difficult for persons with AS/HFA to deal with idioms ("We can't go outside; it's raining cats and dogs"), sarcasm ("oh, great!" when a mistake is made), and subtleties ("do you *want* to go to Time Out?").

The implication of these receptive communication problems is that *visual information should be used to supplement or substitute for verbal information.* Visual information as a supplement is always appropriate; it is particularly important as a substitute for verbal language when the person with AS/HFA is becoming agitated or overwhelmed. Rather than follow the impulse to explain the situation or try to reason with the person with AS/HFA when he is distressed, *the most helpful first response is to stop talking.* Then find a visual way to convey information that will help the person with AS/HFA understand the situation, or options that may help him to calm down and feel more in control.

For most people with AS/HFA, written information is usually the most practical form of visual information. However, in certain situations and for young children or some individuals, other forms of visual information such as photographs, pictures, drawings, or other symbols (e.g., a red circle with diagonal line, meaning "do not") may also be useful.

Written information can contain various types of content:

■   A list of activities (i.e. a schedule). Example: "school, snack, haircut, music lesson, homework, supper."
■   Directions for chores and daily routines, either singly or in a list. Example: "Put dirty clothes in hamper, Take a shower, Shave, Get dressed, Eat breakfast."
■   Directions for calming down in a distressing situation. Example: "Take a deep breath and follow me out of the cafeteria."
■   A list of choices (particularly helpful when the person is upset). Example: "Draw with markers OR Sit in rocking chair OR Listen to relaxation tape."

- A list of rules. Example: "Raise your hand and wait for teacher to say your name before answering questions." "Get permission from your supervisor before leaving the building."
- A list of strategies. Example: "Ask another student for help. Ask the teacher or assistant for help. Sit patiently and think about your ideas until the teacher calls your name. If you feel tense, take 10 slow, deep breaths."
- Reminders: Examples: "Put your paper in the red basket on the teacher's desk when you have finished." "After you finish your paper, read a book until everyone else has finished." "Take your math book with you to math class." "Turn on dishwasher before leaving for work."
- Explanations of social situations using "social stories." The social story technique was developed by Carol Gray, a public school teacher of students with AS/HFA. A social story is a series of brief, written sentences which explain events or situations in the person's life that are causing difficulty, on the assumption that the difficulty is probably due to lack of information or cognitive confusion. Examples might be:

  - "Why we wash our hands before eating"
  - "Why we put on different clothes every day"
  - "Why we stand in lines"
  - "Why we go to school"
  - "Why it is good not to be first all of the time"
  - "What happens at a birthday party/church service/car wash/ barber"
  - "Why we have a babysitter/substitute teacher/fire drill/ snowstorm"
  - "Why schedules sometimes change"

Social stories must always be individually written for each student, because each individual's areas of confusion and ways of understanding are different. They are usually written in the first person. Social stories should contain a high proportion of sentences that describe and explain the situation or describe others' perspectives (such as "most children feel happy when they put on clean clothes" or "most people think they look better if they wear different clothes on different days. They usually wait at least 2 days before wearing the same clothes again"). A smaller proportion of the sentences contain directions to the youngster (such as "After I wear an outfit to school, I will wait a few days before I wear it again"). Carol Gray recommends a "social story ratio" of 0–1 directive sentences for every 2–5 descriptive or perspective sentences. Social stories for young children are generally brief, while those for older students and adults can be somewhat longer, as the concepts that may need to be explained (such as dating, driving privileges, financial responsibility) are more complex.

More information is available in *The Social Story Book*, which can be ordered from Future Horizons, Inc. 721 W. Abram Street, Arlington, Texas 76013; telephone (800) 489-0727; or http://www.futurehorizons.com. Additional information is also available from the Gray Center for Social Learning and Understanding; telephone (616) 667-2396 or email gcenter@gateway.net.

2. In addition to difficulties with verbal language, people with AS/HFA generally have some degree of difficulty understanding and using nonverbal elements of communication such as facial expression, body language, and tone of voice. Very often people with AS/HFA do not interpret these signals in the standard ways they are interpreted in our culture. Further, their facial expressions and manner of speaking may be misinterpreted by others around them. The implication of this is that *explanations and instructions should be explicit rather than implied and observers should not assume that they can interpret the feelings of the person with AS/HFA based on his body language.* Facial expressions that might be interpreted as a "knowing smile," smirk, or look of defiance might not accurately reflect these feelings or thoughts on the part of the person with AS/HFA. It is important to remember that the symbolic aspects of facial expressions and body posture may not be understood or appropriately used by the person with AS/HFA.

3. "Behavior problems" in people with AS/HFA (such as breaking rules, tantrums, and noncompliance with directions) are generally the result of misunderstanding, over-stimulation, or compulsivity secondary to AS/HFA, rather than deficiencies or deliberate attempts to obtain a certain consequence. For example, a person might break into line in a busy cafeteria because he does not understand the unwritten,

unspoken system of lining up. He may have a tantrum in the cafeteria because there is too much noise, movement, and smell. He may refuse to leave the cafeteria because he still has food on his plate or because the clock is broken and is not showing the time that he usually leaves.

The circumstances underlying problematic behaviors are generally more powerful in causing and maintaining the behavior than are typical consequences (such as attention from adults or peers, tangible rewards, etc.). Therefore, *interventions should focus on modification of circumstances, rather than consequences.* Typical behavior management plans, such as loss of privileges, time out, etc., are often of limited usefulness, although sometimes reward and response cost systems can be a helpful adjunct to other intervention plans. For example, instead of responding to a temper tantrum by withdrawing privileges or assigning extra work, it is more effective to analyze the situation that led up to the tantrum. By doing this, one or more of the following factors will generally be found: the individual

- was unclear about what he was supposed to do
- found the task too difficult or unstructured
- was experiencing a sensory overload
- was interrupted and not allowed to finish an activity that he was used to completing

Introducing a punishment or withdrawal of privileges into this type of situation is likely to escalate the emotional distress, rather than reduce it. Remember that intense cognitive confusion that leads to acting out can occur even in persons with extremely high intelligence. Rather than punishing it, avoid it through the use of reliable schedules, preparation for changes, and visual cues about expectations.

4. Sizing up situations and understanding quickly what should be done are not well-developed skills in persons with AS/HFA (Klin et al., 1995). *Persons with AS/HFA need additional information to know how to function in most settings.* In concrete terms, this means that they need to be told what to do and how to act. They need to have this information communicated to them explicitly (using visual means, as described above). They function much better in structured settings

with clear schedules, routines, rules, and physical organization of toys/materials than they do in unstructured or loosely structured settings. Social stories are also a helpful strategy for explaining to individuals what to expect and how to behave in various situations (such as a crowded store, a family gathering, a sibling's recital, Halloween, an airport, etc.).

5. While learning facts, vocabulary, computer skills, and other concrete knowledge may come relatively easily to people with AS/HFA, the nature and connections among feelings, interpersonal events, nonverbal communication, and social expectations are generally much more difficult to understand. *Individuals with AS/HFA need repeated, explicit information about social and emotional topics.* Even basic behavioral expectations, such as looking at someone who is talking, taking turns in a conversation, or saying goodbye before walking away may need to be explained, practiced, prompted, and praised many more times than with a typically developing person. Similarly, the names of feelings, the facial expressions that accompany them, and the effect of behavior on others' feelings may have to be taught explicitly and repeatedly. Attwood (1998) suggests teaching each emotion separately, both in terms of recognizing it in others and expressing it with socially appropriate body language and vocabulary.

A good resource for social/emotional materials is Childswork/ Childsplay (telephone (800) 962-1141), a mail-order firm specializing in books and games about feelings and behavior. An extensive list of materials for teaching about social and emotional topics is contained in Attwood's excellent book *Asperger's syndrome: A guide for parents and professionals*, available from Future Horizons (800 489-0727).

6. Many people with AS/HFA have atypical sensory systems. Many are hypersensitive to sound and/or to tactile stimulation, so that they are stressed in noisy environments, dislike certain clothing textures, don't like to be touched, etc. Other individuals seem to crave specific sensory experiences, such as being squeezed, swinging, listening to music, seeing rows of numbers or toys, etc. A general principle of intervention is to *respect the sensory needs and sensitivities of the individual with AS/HFA.* This often means reducing the amount of

stimulation in problematic situations. At times sensory integration treatment from qualified occupational therapists may be helpful in modifying the individual's atypical sensory processing patterns. But if this is not possible or has not yet happened, it is important to realize how strong and involuntary the individual's sensory patterns are. Rather than seeing these as behavior problems to be modified, they need to be accepted (and channeled into socially tolerable forms if necessary).

Excellent resources for understanding and coping with the sensory sensitivities of people with AS/HFA include *The Out of Sync Child: Recognizing and Coping with Sensory Integration Disorder* by Carol Kranowitz (available from Penguin Putnam, (800) 788-6262) and the chapter on sensory sensitivity in Attwood's *Asperger's Syndrome* book.

7. Since AS/HFA is a chronic, neurologically-based developmental disorder, eliminating all of its manifestations is not going to be possible, and both the individual and the family will be extremely frustrated and unhappy if this is set at a goal. *An important part of intervention is knowing when not to intervene.* There are some elements of the individual's personality and behavior that should probably be accepted and left alone. Interventions are best directed toward goals that are both important and reachable. Sometimes it is hard to know what is reachable until you try. But after reasonable trials to eliminate behaviors such as body-rocking, occasional hand-flapping, lengthy discourses on obscure topics, etc., it may be appropriate to accept the fact that these behaviors are going to happen and probably bring the individual pleasure, and to channel them toward private places and specified times.

8. A final general principle is that the *special interests of people with AS/HFA can and should be appreciated and seen as strengths, rather than simply as symptoms.* Creative teachers and parents can often find ways to link these special interests to other skills the student will need to function in his culture. For example, at young ages beloved figures can be matched, sorted, sequenced, counted, collated, labeled, etc. In later years, written assignments, reading, and even math tasks can incorporate the special topic of interest to the student (for example, writing with good punctuation and spelling about dinosaurs; learning to multiply or divide dinosaurs into packing crates). Adults with AS/HFA can find great personal satisfaction in

working in fields associated with their special interests (such as computers, geography, art).

ADDITIONAL PRINCIPLES OF INTERVENTION

1. *Interventions will be necessary indefinitely.* While the student with AS/HFA has higher intelligence and more skills than individuals with lower functioning autism, AS/HFA is still a significant, life-long developmental disorder. AS/HFA can impair the individual's ability to function in every setting and situation in his/her life. Therefore, consistent support, structure, and modifications must be provided by understanding adults in all situations.

2. *Working with youngsters with AS/HFA is labor-intensive* for clinicians and teachers as well as for parents. Although these students may be served in regular education classes or settings for students with learning disabilities or mild educational handicaps, their service needs are not necessarily less time-consuming or complex than those of lower-functioning students in the autism spectrum. It requires a significant amount of time and thought to design instructional modifications and develop effective behavioral plans, communicate them, implement them consistently, and monitor their continued usefulness. These are not optional services, however; they are necessary for the individual to function. With them, many individuals with AS/HFA can mange beautifully in regular education and vocational settings. Without them, problems often arise. While the specific needs of a child with AS/HFA inevitably change over time (as those of adults may, as well), having special needs never goes away entirely, so no one with AS/HFA should be required to function without special help or modifications of some type.

3. At the time this chapter is being written, it is almost certainly the case that most persons with AS/HFA have spent a significant part of their lives being misunderstood. Similarly, most of their parents have been or felt blamed in some way for their offspring's atypical behaviors. An important part of intervention, therefore, is to *help families learn about AS/HFA and understand that it is a biologically-based*

disorder, not a psychological problem. Through reading about AS/ HFA, talking with other parents, meeting other families, talking with professionals, or in whatever other way(s) they are comfortable, parents need to learn

- that AS/HFA is not their fault
- that the individual's difficulties reflect cognitive confusion and sensory sensitivities rather than poor parenting
- that they can be effective in teaching their offspring and in obtaining needed services

Resources for additional information and support are listed at the end of this chapter. Some families have also found that locating and/or purchasing materials about AS/HFA for teachers, school administrators, and other professionals is appreciated and helpful.

4. *Intervention plans must be coordinated among all caregivers.* Because of the nature of AS/HFA, the world is a confusing place for the individual. Expectations may be unclear, social cues are often missed, events happen unpredictably and for unknown reasons. Given this baseline of confusion, the person with AS/HFA needs his world to be as understandable and predictable as possible. It is not helpful when rules and expectations also differ between parents, between home and school or home and work, among teachers, etc.

It is also important for information about current situations and upcoming events to be available to all caregivers, since the person with AS/HFA needs as much preparation and reassurance as possible. For example, teachers can let parents know about upcoming field trips and projects, parents can alert staff about family events, the individual's health, eating, and sleeping status, etc. Keeping communication flowing is time-consuming, but it is vital for all involved to do so and for someone to take on the responsibility of overseeing the decision-making and communication processes.

A system for communication should be explicitly agreed to among the adults involved. This may take the form of regular telephone calls or voice mail messages, daily notes, a communication notebook that moves with the individual among settings, a central contact person, or other methods that fit a particular set of circumstances.

It is important not to depend on the person with AS/HFA to relay important messages unless it has been established that he/she reliably does so (Moreno, 1991). It is difficult for some youngsters with AS/HFA even to answer questions about their day at school. A technique that has been helpful in developing this skill is the use of a large zip-loc bag that goes back and forth between home and school. In the bag are put "souvenirs" or symbols from important activities, to serve as a concrete, visual focus for talking about events of the day.

5. *Developing interventions for AS/HFA requires an attitude of flexibility* and willingness to individualize planning in creative and unorthodox ways. Developing interventions is also a dynamic process: problems resolve but new issues emerge; the individual with AS/HFA masters new skills and understanding but environmental demands increase; helpful plans are agreed to, but teachers and staff change, etc.

AGE-SPECIFIC INTERVENTIONS

PRESCHOOL-AGE CHILDREN

Bobby was a 4-year-old boy who was brought for evaluation by his parents because he was having behavioral difficulties at his small, private nursery school. His developmental milestones were within normal limits and there were no health concerns. Although he was described as a colicky and very active baby, his behavior and developmental patterns were not thought by his parents to be problematic until they attempted to have him participate in various group childcare activities. At age $2\frac{1}{2}$ he was asked to discontinue group babysitting at the Y while his mother swam, at age 3 he was unsuccessful at story time at the library, at age $3\frac{1}{4}$ he was asked to leave a part-time daycare center after two months, and during the course of the psychological evaluation, the director of his nursery school decided that he could no longer be served there because of the behavioral disruptions that he caused. Before this happened, however, the psychologist was able to observe him in school.

He was observed to wander between activities, often knocking over other children's materials. It seemed as though he liked to see things fly through the air or fall, and did not realize that he was hurting, frightening, or annoying other children. While he did speak several times to other children ("look at me, Mary"), he did not enter into their conversations with each other. At one point he said to another child, "Susie, you know what? We have a fan that squeaks because it needs WD-40." This child did not respond, and apparently was not interested in this topic. The parents reported that Bobby had long been fascinated with fans: he insisted on going to the fan section of the home supply store, he watched fans in restaurants, and he had a large collection of toy fans and old fan parts. At age 4, his WPPSI-R Verbal IQ was 127, Performance IQ 110, Full Scale IQ 122.

Diagnoses of possible AS/HFA are beginning to be made at the preschool level. Difficulties these children have are generally first noted in group childcare settings, where their developmental differences are more obvious than at home. The difficulties for which preschool children end up being referred to psychologists are usually behavioral non-compliance or disruptive behavior that can escalate into temper tantrums.

The most basic intervention at this stage is a complete developmental evaluation, ideally by a team that includes a developmental pediatrician or child psychiatrist, a speech/language clinician who includes assessment of pragmatics and auditory processing in the evaluation, an occupational therapist experienced with sensory integration dysfunction, and a psychologist with a developmental/behavioral orientation. As part of the evaluation, a thorough explanation for parents of the AS/HFA diagnosis, resources for obtaining additional information, and information or consultation for the childcare providers (if the parents want this) should be provided. This information should be presented with compassion, honesty, and sensitivity to the fact that the diagnosis may be emotionally wrenching for the family (Shea, 1984, 1993).

Behavior problems, as described above, are generally caused by cognitive confusion, sensory overload, or compulsive behaviors.

Therefore, for preschool children the following suggestions are generally appropriate:

- Talk less. Give one direction at a time.
- Talk more slowly.
- Shorten your statements emphasizing key words.
- Use pictures in addition to words to provide information to the child. Their most important uses are in preparing the child for transitions to new activities or taking the child through activities he/she does not enjoy.
- Structure the child's day with adult-directed activities and predictable routines.
- Try to arrange the child's environment to limit sensory stresses (e.g., noisy places, disliked foods or clothing).
- Teach simple, structured social games with an adult first, then include another child in the play. Provide adult supervision and support to guide play with typically developing peers.
- Rather than trying to eliminate the child's strong, narrow interests, incorporate them into a range of activities in a productive way.

SCHOOL-AGE CHILDREN

Joey was an 8-year-old boy who was in 2nd grade, having repeated Kindergarten because of "social immaturity." He had never been diagnosed with a specific developmental problem, and he was placed in a regular class with no special services. He was referred to the school psychologist because of behavioral outbursts in his classroom and in the cafeteria. Standardized testing revealed high average intelligence and adequate academic achievement, except for large, immature handwriting. He had particular strengths in decoding words, and had been observed reading the mail on the teacher's desk. Behavior checklists completed by his parents and teachers were elevated on scales reflecting cognitive and disruptive behavior problems and attention span, although he was described by his teachers as a generally quiet boy except for his outbursts. These were becoming more frequent, and he was beginning to complain about going to school. He did not have any friends, although some of the girls in the class were protective of him. During free time at school, he generally chose to use the computer or to draw pictures of electric power grids. During recess he wandered around the perimeter of the playground.

Social Issues

Making friends and behaving appropriately in social situations are areas of significant difficulty for children with AS/HFA. Children with AS/HFA do not pick up the unstated rules of social interactions without explicit instruction and practice. Learning social skills should be a part of the IEP for almost all school-age children with AS/HFA. Skills that may need to be addressed include:

- waiting
- taking turns at being first
- taking turns making decisions about what to play/do
- joining in a conversation or activity with other children
- taking turns in a conversation
- working/playing quietly
- accepting not winning

(This list of social interaction skills was adapted from *Helping People with Autism Manage Their Behavior* by Nancy Justin Dalrymple. This booklet is part of an excellent series, *Functional Programming for People with Autism* published by the Indiana Resource Center for Autism, Indiana University, Institute for the Study of Developmental Disabilities, 2853 East Tenth Street, Bloomington, Indiana 47408-2601; telephone (812) 855-6508).

Students with AS/HFA can learn to understand social expectations better, particularly if these are made concrete and visual, and if they are repeatedly demonstrated, discussed, practiced, and rewarded. As noted above, the social stories technique of Carol Gray is one excellent method for explaining to students with AS/HFA how the social world operates. Gray has also developed a technique for talking with students with AS/HFA about problematic or confusing social situations they have experienced. This technique, called "Comic Strip Conversations," involves drawing the people in the situation and their words, thoughts, and feelings. The use of drawings takes advantage of visual means to communicate about abstract, verbal ideas (such as interrupting, keeping angry thoughts unspoken, interpreting facial expressions as well as spoken words). Different symbols are used to illustrate what was said vs. what was meant, and different colors are used to illustrate the feelings of the various characters in the interaction (for example, green = happy, friendly; red = unfriendly, bad). This technique is helpful in identifying where the student's confusion lies by helping him to analyze social interactions. Further, the underlying assumptions, complexities, and nuances of the situation can be explained and taught in this visual way. More information about Comic Strip Conversations is available from Future Horizons: (800) 489-0727 or from The Gray Center for Social Learning and Understanding: (616) 667-2396.

Another technique for making social relationships and corresponding social behavior visual, in order to make this complex topic more understandable, is described in Attwood's book, *Asperger's syndrome: A guide for parents and professionals.* The term he uses is Circle of Friends (which is different from the Circle of Friends process of supplementing the support and guidance from parents with that from a larger set of friends and community helpers). The technique Attwood describes involves drawing a series of concentric circles, with the individual with AS/HFA in the center, to illustrate the progression outward from close family, extended family and close friends, neighbors and friendly acquaintances, professional helpers, strangers, etc. This visual information about degree of social relationship can assist in teaching the individual appropriate social behavior (for example, who can be hugged, who should not be teased, etc.).

Teaching social skills might need to begin with an adult's working with the child with AS/HFA, but practicing social skills by definition has to be done with peers. Therefore, some of this work must be done at school or other group settings. Skills should first be taught in structured situations, meaning that activities have been designed by the adult(s) to make use of the social skill(s) being worked on. In school settings this can be done in various settings, including the regular classroom or a special education class, in speech/language or occupational therapy, in sessions with the guidance counselor, or in other structured settings selected by the IEP team.

After the skills have been practiced under controlled conditions with an adult, one or two typically developing children could be brought into the activity to allow for more natural practice. Later, gentle reminders can be used with the student with AS/HFA in less structured settings, such as recess, the playground, cafeteria, etc.

Related to teaching social skills and behaviors is teaching children with AS/HFA to play some of the same games as their classmates. In some classes, this can be as simple as teaching the student to play board games and card games that other students his/her age enjoy. In other situations, it may be possible for a teacher to analyze and simplify the activities of the other students, so that the child with AS/HFA can join in. For example, free-form games with balls could be organized into catch, throwing to a goal, bouncing contests, dodge ball, etc. Random running could be re-structured into tag. Children could be encouraged to sit together and color different parts of a large picture, or work together on a complex, multi-piece puzzle. Additional ideas are contained in the manual and videotape "Integrated Play Groups" by Pam Wolfberg, available from California Research Institute, 612 Font Boulevard, San Francisco, CA 94132; telephone (415) 338-7847; Fax (415) 338-6121.

In order to help children with poor social skills fit in better at school, it can be very helpful for teachers or parents to explain AS/HFA to other students in the child's class (at a time that he is not there). Parents of the other students may be able to guide their children to be kind and understanding if they are given information about the child with AS/HFA. (See the following example, adapted from work by Lisa Lieberman.) Also, Carol Gray has developed a lesson plan for classmates, called The Sixth Sense, which enables them to experience the confusion and distress that can be caused by not having an understanding of the social communication among classmates. This is available in

Taming the Recess Jungle, which can be ordered from Future Horizons, Inc. (800) 489-0727.

August 30, 2001

To Elm Street Elementary School 2nd Grade Parents,

Our son, Johnny Jones, has just enrolled at Elm Street for the year, after spending 1st grade at Greenway. We are writing to introduce ourselves and to welcome your support in making this transition a smooth one for Johnny.

Johnny is $7\frac{1}{2}$, a happy, loving little boy who wants very much to have friends. He loves music, being physically active, and playing on the computer. He also likes to read, and he understands math concepts within a normal range of expectations for beginning second graders.

Johnny is unique in that he has Asperger Syndrome, which is sometimes called high functioning autism. For many, that term brings up a stereotyped image of a child rocking in a corner, unable to communicate with the world. This is far from the case with our son and many others with the same diagnosis. Asperger Syndrome comes from a difference in brain functioning that affects how Johnny learns about the world around him and how he communicates to others. It is a neurological disorder, complicated by a difficulty in screening out sensory input (sound, touch, small visual detail, taste, etc.). When he is overstimulated or confused he might do things that can be difficult to understand, including such non-aggressive behaviors as flapping his hands when he is excited, leaving a room temporarily if there is too much stimulation, taking a long time to process what is said to him before answering, and talking too loudly or too much.

Asperger Syndrome also includes very literal, concrete interpretations of what is being said. This actually leads to some very humorous things done and said in total ignorance, adding to his charm. Johnny makes people laugh, and often doesn't understand what is funny, but he takes genuine pleasure in eliciting laughter in others. Because Johnny looks so "normal" physically, it takes a while for people to understand his social and educational difficulties. He may sometimes appear rude, because of his difficulty grasping social subtleties and the time it takes his brain to process what is being said to him.

We are moving Johnny to Elm Street now because we feel it is important for him to go to school in his own neighborhood. Our goal is to help him connect with children who live close by. Your child can be an important part of making him feel welcome at Elm Street. We also believe that your child will benefit from having Johnny in the class. Johnny will have an instructional assistant in the classroom, whose job it is to help him function as independently as possible. This means that the assistant is often available to assist the teacher in other ways, which is, of course, a benefit to other children in the class. More importantly, we feel that people like Johnny have much to teach others about honoring diversity, and about the richness that comes from being exposed to people who are different.

We hope this letter helps to inform you, in a positive way, about our son's disability. Please remember that above all else there is a boy in there who loves to learn, wants to follow the rules (once he understands what is expected), who needs to feel that he belongs, and who wants very much to have friends like any other child.

Johnny loves to have children over to play. He has a very inviting room with a dual-control Nintendo, lots of action figures, and plenty of room for little race cars. If you think your child might enjoy coming over to play, we welcome you to come along too, and meet us. We also invite you to call with any concerns or questions. Thanks for taking the time to read this letter.

Sincerely,
Jim and Sally Jones
321 Elm Street
Centerville, California
Telephone: 555-1234

Some teachers and families also set up a "buddy system" or network of children who are asked to include and help the student with AS/HFA, and who are reinforced by teachers for doing so. Teachers can also

- set up a class atmosphere in which teasing and bullying are not permitted
- use alternate ways to divide into teams or select partners, so that the student with AS/HFA is not always the last one chosen
- design cooperative learning groups and games in which the special talents/interests of the student with AS/HFA are useful and appreciated by other students (for example: sophisticated vocabulary, good sight word or spelling skills, knowledge of facts in specific areas can help the team win)
- use classroom situations to teach about feelings and interpersonal relations (for example, how it feels to be teased, ignored, interrupted, left out of a game, stared at, criticized, etc.). Some of these topics might help the student with AS/HFA understand his/her classmates better, and some might help the classmates appreciate the effect of their behavior on the student with AS/HFA.

Students with AS/HFA may be eager to know how to fit into activities with their classmates, or they may prefer to spend time alone engaged in their special pursuits (such as studying road maps or drawing flags). In either situation, engaging them in structured games (such as card games or board games) with other children is recommended.

Sometimes parents can work on social skills in home and community settings. They may need help in identifying the skill(s) to be worked on, communicating it to the student, structuring situations effectively, and providing feedback to their child. Some parents have selected peer models for their children, explained AS/HFA to them, and even paid them to take their child into the community or include the child with AS/HFA in outings, neighborhood games, etc. The friendships of youngsters with AS/HFA may be more activity-based and less communicative than friendships of other children, but they are usually very meaningful to the people involved. Parents may need to modify their hopes for standard popularity in order to help their child spend enjoyable time with peers he feels comfortable with. This may mean other children with special needs, even significant disabilities, which may not be the peer group parents had hoped for. However, for the child with AS/HFA to feel that he has some true "friends" is extremely important and pleasurable.

Academic Issues

Modified Expectations and Procedures

In all autism spectrum disorders, skills are widely scattered, so that talents in one area do not necessarily predict talents in other areas. This is even true for tasks that appear to be closely related. For example,

- a student who can read well for facts might have difficulty with making interpretations and inferences from the reading
- a student who can carry out complex computations might be unable to make change, etc. (Moreno, 1991; Williams, 1995)
- a student with good ideas and adequate organizational skills might produce limited written work or might resist all writing assignments because of poor fine motor skills which result in messy handwriting and an aching hand
- a student with excellent sight reading abilities might have poor reading comprehension.

Therefore, expectations and assignments for students with AS/HFA must be individualized. Every class assignment has potential pitfalls for the student with AS/HFA, which again points out why these students require on-going modifications and planning. Because of these students' good intelligence, peak skills, and typical appearance, it is easy for teachers and parents to forget the multiple cognitive challenges the students face on a daily basis. Too many children with AS/HFA, even after they have been diagnosed and identified, have been thought of as unmotivated, disobedient, uncooperative, or manipulative, when it is far more likely that they have not understood or been able to meet expectations in school.

Among the modifications that students with AS/HFA often need are:

- additional time on tests because of organizational, attention, and handwriting problems
- reduced written homework assignments for the same reasons (Williams, 1995 also points out that struggles over homework can increase the stress on families, which may be a legitimate reason to limit the amount of homework assigned)
- permission/encouragement to dictate work to a parent or other adult
- modified testing arrangements, testing in a separate room, oral testing, writing on the question sheet, multiple choice or circle the answer format, testing that uses the same visual schedule/directions/check off system used throughout the student's school day, etc.
- modified grading system, based on IEP goals rather than typical class goals

Such modifications need to be thought through in the initial IEP meeting and may need to be modified in subsequent meetings, since there may be serious consequences of standardized test scores or grades in terms of promotion/retention or documentation of a need for modifications in the future (e.g. when taking college entrance tests).

Written vs. Auditory Information

Extensive use of written information is almost always an effective strategy for helping students with AS/HFA. Spoken language is a source of stimulation that can be disturbing to these youngsters. Research studies repeatedly demonstrate the difficulties these students have in understanding complex language and the overstimulation language can cause. Keeping language simple and minimizing its emphasis as the primary classroom teaching modality is an important way to help students with AS/HFA. Writing down important information, rather than always delivering it orally, can lead to more effective communication and fewer adverse side effects from overstimulation. Written language is also more concrete and better suited to the slower language processing that is frequently associated with this disability. For classroom discussions, written information can be provided as handouts, worksheets, study questions, written lists of directions, etc. Visual aids, such as maps, charts, pictures, and objects, are also extremely helpful for these students when a class involves academic concepts.

Organizational Strategies

Students with AS/HFA will also need strategies for organizing their school materials, classwork, and assignments. Organization difficulties are among the most handicapping of the problems associated with AS/HFA because they interfere with the initiation, performance, and generalization of most tasks. Organizational strategies that increase predictability and clarity of the tasks are especially effective for the AS/HFA group because they enable them to utilize their considerable skills in productive and meaningful ways.

There are two levels of written organizational systems that should generally be provided to students with AS/HFA. The first relates to the sequence of activities during the day, and the second to the steps of each individual activity or work task.

Daily Schedule. A written daily schedule is an important support for students with AS/HFA, because it enables the student to predict the expectations of the situation. Increasing predictability is essential for students with AS/HFA because class schedules, especially in middle school and high school, can be imprecise, confusing, and pressured, and therefore anxiety-provoking.

Daily schedules should be individualized for each student to maximize understanding and flexibility. For example:

Student 1:
   Math
   PE
   Language Arts

Student 2:
    8:55 Get book and folder for math class out of backpack
    9:00 When the bell rings, go to math class
    9:45 Go to locker and get clothes for PE
    9:55 Go to PE
    10:45 Go to locker, put away gym clothes, and get books and
        folders for Language Arts and Spanish

Even though Student 2 is in high school and is able to read and understand at a high school level, the schedule is helpful because it arranges for each activity to be checked off after it occurs and provides a visual reminder of what activities will be done and in what sequence each day. Student 1 is probably younger and does not have a clear concept of time. This student's language is also more limited, so the limited number of words on the schedule reflects the amount of information that she is able to process with total comprehension.

Individual schedules should be designed to meet the needs of individual students. Students might use half-day or full-day schedules, depending on their age and overall level of functioning and understanding. The schedules can be handwritten, typed, computer generated, or written on a write-on/wipe-off board. Students should manipulate their schedule, as they complete specific activities, by crossing items off, making check marks, erasing, turning completed items over, or whatever is satisfying and meaningful to them. The important point is that they manipulate the schedule and can see that they are making progress, finishing something, and moving toward the end of the school day. The schedule could also include standard reminders such as "bring a pencil," "check the board for homework assignment," "turn in your homework before beginning classswork," etc.

In addition to helping with organization and predictability, schedules also help with flexibility, because individual items can appear anywhere on a schedule, and whenever changes are necessary, they can be inserted clearly for the student to see immediately and understand. Thus, the schedule might change, but whatever is on the schedule is always reliable.

Clearly, such schedules need to be carefully thought out and individualized for the student's individualized organizational needs.

Again, developing these is time-consuming, but can make the difference between a successful, calm student and one who is confused,
late, unprepared for class, and stressed.

Organizational Systems for Individual Activities. In addition to
schedules that facilitate movement from one activity to the next, students with AS/HFA may need help while they are working at specific
activities in order to stay focused and to understand the expectations.
Therefore, the second level of written directions is for individual activities, which can include academic tasks, preparing for work, classroom
chores, lesson preparation, or any other classroom activities that
require the sequential organizational abilities that are difficult for students with AS/HFA.

An organizational system for work tasks should communicate to
students four essential pieces of information:

- What work or activity needs to be done
- How much needs to be done
- How they can see that they are progressing and when they
  will be finished
- What will happen after their work/activity is finished

Work systems serve several important functions. First, they specify
exactly what the students are supposed to do in the kind of clear, direct,
visual, and concrete way that is most meaningful to them. Second, work
systems help keep students focused by highlighting the tasks at hand
and the location where the student should be in completing each task.
Third, these systems also help with organization and sequencing,
chronic problems for all students with AS/HFA. Finally, there is an
important motivational aspect to the process each students go through of
checking off components of their tasks as they complete them, and seeing exactly how much they have accomplished and what is left to do.

Work systems should be individualized according to the student's
needs and the particular tasks, which allows the teacher to make
instructions more concrete and specific for their students with

AS/HFA. Written or other visual directions are more likely to be successful if they are presented to students individually at their workspace, rather than written on the blackboard.

For students who do not need step-by step directions, a commonly used work system is a series of color/coded or numbered folders, each one containing a specific assignment. For example, the student's schedule directs him or her to a classroom or workspace where there are three folders to be completed. This answers the questions "What work?" and "How much work?" After completing each folder, the student checks it off the list of tasks or puts the folder in a finished basket. This answers the question "How do I know I am progressing toward being finished?" Then the work system or the student's schedule indicates what the next activity is.

For some students it will be necessary to have in each folder specific work assignments described in detail. For example:

- Take out your Language Arts book
- Take out a sheet of paper
- Turn to page 84
- Write the answers to questions 1–10 on your paper
- Write your name at the top of the paper
- Put your paper in the green folder on (teacher's) desk
- Sit at your desk and read your reading book until (teacher) calls on you

For a younger student a series of instructions can be listed next to any activity. For example, if the daily task is to feed the class's pet hamster, the list could indicate pouring a specific quantity of food in a cup, placing the cup in the cage, filling up the water bottle, and putting the food away. As with the academic folders, the student checks off each of these activities as it is completed.

Visual Clarity. It is helpful for most students with AS/HFA to have assignments spaced generously on the page and for each step to be visually clear, since the more information placed on a single page, the more difficult it is for students to sort out what is essential.

- Small print or double column reading assignments can be made much easier by spreading out the text, typing an adaptation, or using a version designed for visually impaired students.
- For any assignment, reducing the number of items on a page, using larger print, spreading items out, highlighting relevant concepts, or clarifying where answers are to be written and how many answers are required can be useful strategies.
- Visual models of what answers should look like are also helpful.

Organization of Materials. The organization of materials can also simplify the lives of these students and result in more successful academic performances. Students with AS/HFA may need the following types of support at school:

- Teacher supervision in cleaning out desk or locker regularly
- Assignment sheets either prepared or supervised by the teacher
- Duplicate books at home (so that the student does not need to carry all books home or remember which ones are needed each night)
- Use of a different colored folder for each subject, with one side for the assignment sheet and related materials and one side for completed work to be turned in
- Organizing the student's belongings at home for transport to and from school
- Organizing home and school desks so that papers, pencils, reference books, calculators, and other materials have a specific place, in order to reduce the amount of wasted time spent on looking for materials
- Clearly labeling textbooks and other materials to reduce wasted time off task

The physical structure of the classroom and each individual's work area can either promote or detract from a student's ability to work effectively. Writings of adults with autism (Grandin, 1995;

Williams, 1988) describe sensory distractions that interfere with their concentration and ability to focus. Stimulation is not only distracting, but can actually increase anxiety and trigger behavioral disturbances. Temple Grandin has talked extensively about the Squeeze Machine that she developed to provide herself with a very calm and nonstimulating escape from everyday noises and visual distractions.

Organizing physical space to minimize the negative impact of classroom stimulation is an important component of the Structured Teaching approach. To the extent possible, furniture and classroom space should be arranged so that students with AS/HFA are not bombarded with any more stimulation than is necessary. Preferential seating close to teaching areas is encouraged so that teachers can monitor student progress and so that the student is close to where the instruction is occurring and less likely to be distracted by interfering stimuli. Many students with AS/HFA benefit from having their own independent work area or office desk-like arrangement; a special desk separated from the general classroom by a divider or bookcase can be extremely helpful. It is also helpful if students are faced away from the noisiest or busiest parts of the classroom. Also, for students with AS/HFA, a quiet area where they can go when their anxiety levels are especially high is another important classroom modification.

Students with AS/HFA may also be very stressed by regular Physical Education classes, where expectations for gross motor coordination are way beyond their level, and peer interactions may be unpleasant or even cruel. Adaptive Physical Education or alternative activities during PE may be necessary.

Additional suggestions are available in an excellent book *Higher Functioning Adolescents and Adults with Autism: A Teacher's Guide* (Fullerton et al., 1996) available from Pro-Ed (8700 Shoal Creek Boulevard, Austin, Texas 78757-6897; telephone (800) 897-3202; or http://www.proedinc.com).

Behavior Problems and Emotional Issues

A typical behavior problem seen in school-age youngsters with AS/HFA is repetitive questioning or arguing with a teacher. These students can be extremely skilled at "quibbling" about details of directions or rules. For example, "I wasn't running, I was loping," "I didn't hit him, I tapped him," "You didn't say to use a pencil, so I wrote with only my finger," "But I already know these words, so I don't want to write them in sentences," "But I want to be on the computer *now*." Entering into lengthy discussions about these topics is non-productive. More effective techniques include

- written schedules that can simply be pointed to
- written rules (including a rule about arguing about the rules and a rule that all behaviors in a general category are covered by a general rule)
- written dialogue with the student about his feelings and concerns, which may be more calming and comprehensible for him than a verbal discussion
- a specific time of the day to discuss questions or concerns. Students can be referred back to their schedules whenever they have concerns at other times of the day

For students who have difficulty staying on task, it sometimes helps for the teacher and student to agree on a nonverbal signal the teacher can use to indicate "please get back to work" (Williams, 1995).

Emotional coping and relaxation skills can be useful for older individuals with AS/HFA (Attwood, 1998; Moreno, 1991; Williams, 1995). These skills include slow, deep breathing; counting; tensing and relaxing muscles, visualizing pleasant scenes; going to a quiet, "safe place" in school to calm down; and going to see a designated "special helper" such as the guidance counselor or resource teacher at times of stress. Attwood also describes the following possible interventions to help reduce anxiety or anger:

- solitude
- soothing music
- massage
- distraction toward a favorite or successful activity
- thinking positive thoughts
- physical exercise
- medication

- Cognitive Behavioral Therapy for anxiety. This is an intervention by a mental health professional that can be helpful in situations of intense anxiety, sometimes accompanied by phobias or obsessive-compulsive behaviors. There are several variations of this technique. In one, the individual is helped to become desensitized to the source of the anxiety by gradually visualizing or experiencing it while remaining relaxed through the use of competing visualizations or behaviors such as deep breathing and/or imagining a pleasant, happy situation. In a more cognitive, abstract version, the individual is helped to analyze and gain cognitive control of his fears and sources of anxiety, and provided with alternate thoughts/interpretations of anxiety-arousing situations.

Transition to Adulthood

By junior high school, parents and teachers should begin thinking about the vocational capabilities of the student with AS/HFA and planning IEP goals accordingly. Ideally, the special interests of the student with AS/HFA can be incorporated in future educational or vocational plans (such as higher education in history, computer technology, or science for students with fascinations with some aspect of these areas). Parents and teachers must also be realistic about the areas of weakness of the student with AS/HFA (generally social skills, motor skills, and ability to handle multiple sensory input simultaneously) because jobs that depend on these skills are likely to be difficult and unpleasant for the person with AS/HFA (Klin et al., 1995).

Also by junior high school, parents should seriously consider talking with their child about the diagnosis of AS/HFA. Many parents are reluctant to do so, because they are worried that the child will feel that "there is something wrong with him." But in fact the child is already living with the effects and problems of AS/HFA, without the benefits of understanding why he or she has certain difficulties, knowing that it is no one's fault, and knowing that there are other people with similar profiles and problems. It is frequently a great relief to people with AS/HFA to have a name for their pattern of behavior, skills, and difficulties. While it may pain parents to accept and use the "label" of AS/HFA, doing so with their youngster and helping the youngster talk about feeling different or lonely can be a loving, supportive act on their part, and a major contribution to the child's future mental health and adjustment. A suggested social story-type initial explanation of AS/HFA is contained in the appendix. Another excellent resource for explaining AS/HFA to youngsters is "What Does It Mean to Me?" by Catherine Faherty, available from Future Horizons (800 489-0727).

ADULTS

Tre was a 19-year-old man with undiagnosed AS/HFA who had graduated from high school the year before he was brought for evaluation by his mother. He had taken several courses at a community college, but had dropped them before completing them. He was living at home and was dependent on his mother and older brother for transportation, which he resented. He indicated that he was planning to go to a "good college" but could not describe what the application process was or what he wanted to study. He also wanted to get his own apartment, but his mother indicated that he rarely helped with chores around the house and that she even had to remind him to shower, brush his teeth, etc. He periodically made friends through the youth group at church, but eventually they tended to stop calling him and began making excuses to hang up when he called them, which was very disappointing and confusing to him. He generally continued trying to call them, leading one young woman to have a block put on her phone for calls from his number.

The range of skills and needs of adults with AS/HFA is very wide. While some at this end of the autism spectrum might need ongoing help in achieving stable adult functioning, others can function adequately without special support, being considered perhaps slightly "quirky" in their personal and vocational lives. It seems likely that the earlier the intervention to help the youngster with AS/HFA understand social/emotional interactions and be successful in school, the better the eventual adult outcome will be. Part of the intervention plan for older students and young adults may be teaching them to design and implement their own plans for support and organization, so that they know when and where they learn/work best, what form of communication is most effective for them, how to ask for help and additional information, etc. In many cases, supportive and practical counseling from professionals familiar with AS/HFA can be very important. Other families may need to think about financial support and/or some degree of supervision throughout the person's life. Moreno (1991) also suggests that family members might choose to inform community workers (such as police, hospital emergency room, etc.) about the special patterns of their family member with AS/HFA. In addition, the decision might be made to inform employers, roommates, clergy, etc.

RESEARCH LITERATURE

Experimental research on interventions for AS/HFA is quite scarce. Koegel and Frea (1993) reported a multiple baseline intervention targeting various social behaviors of two youngsters with high functioning autism. The dependent variables were facial expression and affect, nonverbal mannerisms (such as rubbing objects or moving arms inappropriately), perseveration of topic, intensity of voice volume, and eye gaze. Subjects were first taught to discriminate inappropriate from appropriate behaviors (demonstrated by the clinician). Then they monitored themselves and recorded successful emission of only appropriate behaviors during specific time periods, which were gradually lengthened. The reinforcer was the opportunity to play video games. Targeted behaviors responded quickly to these contingencies. In addition, there was generalization to as yet untreated behaviors.

Swaggart et al. (1995) presented baseline and post-intervention data for three students with autism (level or degree not specified) for whom written social stories were used to increase various prosocial behaviors and/or decrease aggression. For all three students, stories that essentially described appropriate behaviors and positive consequences were notably successful.

Two studies (Marriage et al., 1989) included an evaluation component in their social skills groups for boys with autism and average intelligence. Williams used cooperative games, role-playing exercises (including analysis of mistakes in role-played scenes), discussions of feelings and associated body language, voice exercises, and practice in clear communication. The intervention techniques used by Marriage et al. included structured games, role-playing and analysis of mistakes, analysis of videotapes (which was not thought to be effective and was discontinued), a "show and tell" activity, cooperative activities (such as cooking together or making collages of pictures of emotions), and homework assignments to practice various skills covered in the group. Pre- and post-intervention data were collected; some statistically significant improvements were found by Williams, but not by Marriage et al.

Hare (1997) described cognitive-behavioral psychotherapy with a 26 year old man with AS/HFA and severe depression. Since cognitive-behavioral therapy for depression focuses on logical analysis and reinterpretation of the client's ideas about his/her current situation, as the foundation for changing problematic feelings and behaviors, it was felt that this approach could be successful with the concrete, logical thinking processes of a person with AS/HFA. During therapy, the client was helped to make connections between events and his feeling states, to identify accurate and reasonable sources of information about events that he otherwise tended to misperceive, and to develop a list of ways to cope with his negative feelings. Much of the work was done in writing, through the use of a journal to record his feelings and associated events. The client's Beck Depression Inventory (BDI) decreased markedly after the 8th treatment session. At 6 months post-treatment, his BDI had increased, although it was not as high as the pre-treatment level.

Debra Kamps and colleagues (Dugan et al., 1995; Garrison-Harrell et al., 1997; Kamps & Kravitz, 1997; Kamps et al., 1994; 1995) have looked at the effect of various instructional strategies and techniques on students with autism (some of whom were high functioning) in regular education classrooms. Peer tutoring, cooperative learning groups, the use of networks of peers trained in social skills, and the use of augmentative communication were all found to be associated with increases in academic engagement, academic skills, and social interaction time.

<hr>

SUMMARY AND CONCLUSION

Individuals with AS/HFA have good potential for learning the skills and knowledge necessary to function as productive, contented adults. To achieve this potential, they require substantial amounts of special instruction, understanding, acceptance, and modification of environmental expectations to accommodate their special needs. Those who teach and care for them must understand the disorder, understand the individual, and be both flexible and thorough in designing plans to accommodate their needs.

<hr>

ADDITIONAL RESOURCES

Asperger Syndrome Coalition of the United States, Inc. website: http://www.asperger.org

Autism Society of America: 800-3-AUTISM or http://www.autism-society.org

Autism Society of NC bookstore: 800 442-2762 or http://www.autismsociety-nc.org

More Advanced Individuals with Autism, Asperger's Syndrome, Pervasive Developmental Disorders: http://www.maapservices.org or 219–662–1311

OASIS website: http://www.udel.edu/bkirby/asperger/

TEACCH website: http://www.teacch.com

Yale AS/HFA project website:
http://www.info.med.yale.edu/chldstdy/autism

<hr>

APPENDIX

<hr>

Outline of a Social Story Explaining AS/HFA

This basic framework can be modified based on a particular individual's situation; some typical characteristics are included in parentheses.

> Everyone has things they are good at and everyone has problems. My mom is good at tennis and cooking. She has a problem with parking the car straight and singing in tune. My dad is good at fixing things. He has a problem with

remembering things he said he would do. I am good at computers and reading and math. I have a problem with (making friends, knowing how to talk to people, getting along with other kids my age, understanding what people mean, understanding social rules that other people seem to understand).

My mom and dad took me to a (doctor, psychologist, therapist, clinic) to find out why I have this problem and how to help me with the problem. My parents learned that the name of my problem is (Asperger Syndrome, AS, autism, HFA). People with (Asperger Syndrome, AS, autism, HFA) have trouble with (making friends, knowing how to talk to people, getting along with other kids my age, understanding what people mean, understanding social rules that other people seem to understand). (Asperger Syndrome, AS, autism, HFA) is not my fault. (Asperger Syndrome, AS, autism, HFA) is not my parents' fault. (Asperger Syndrome, AS, autism, HFA) is no one's fault. I am not sick, I just have a problem. Everyone has some kind of problem, and this one is mine.

(Asperger Syndrome, AS, autism, HFA) makes it hard to (make friends, know how to talk to people, get along with other kids my age, understand what people mean, understand social rules that other people seem to understand). Other problems that are part of (Asperger Syndrome, AS, autism, HFA) are (looking at people when they talk to me, looking at people when I talk to them, talking too loud, doing things with my hands that most people don't do, doing things with my body that most people don't do).

There are ways to help with (making friends, knowing how to talk to people, getting along with other kids my age, understanding what people mean, understanding social rules that other people seem to understand) and with other kinds of problems. My mom/dad can teach me how to do this better. My teacher can teach me how to do this better.

I will work with my mom/dad/teacher to learn how to (make friends, know how to talk to people, get along with other kids my age, understand what people mean, understand social rules that other people seem to understand). That will make me feel better and it will make my mom/dad happy.

Final Thoughts

THE AUTISM SPECTRUM

Many professionals in the field of autism today believe both that autism varies in severity and that autism and normal development are on a continuum. The range of manifestations and degrees of autism is often referred to as the "autism spectrum" (Allen, 1988; Wing, 1988). At one extreme of the autism spectrum are people with severe autism who manifest all of the characteristics to a significant degree. This group usually has significant mental retardation as well. Closer to the normal end of the continuum are people who have the characteristics and behaviors that meet the criteria for a diagnosis of autism, but to a lesser degree in combination with more cognitive, social, communication, and adaptive skills. Even closer to normal, because of average intelligence and more typical language, are people with AS/HFA. PDD-NOS is also an autism spectrum disorder, usually even closer to normal than AS because not all criteria for a diagnosis of autism or AS are met (see Chapter 2 for a discussion of PDD-NOS). It has also been proposed that even closer to the normal end of the continuum are severe learning disabilities (Shea & Mesibov, 1985) or NLD (Rourke, 1989, 1995; Rourke & Tsatsanis, 2000).

DIVISIONS WITHIN THE AUTISM SPECTRUM

For researchers, clinicians, teachers, policy-makers, and families, identification of valid sub-types or meaningful clusters within the broad spectrum of autism could be important.

- Different etiologies and biological mechanisms might have different implications for medical prevention and treatment strategies.
- Significant differences in current presentation and functioning could have implications for educational strategies and related services.
- Clusters of symptoms and behaviors that are associated with a different course or developmental trajectory could enable families better to plan and predict what will be needed for their child in the future.

Over the years, various researchers have attempted to determine whether meaningful sub-types within the autism spectrum exist, and to specify the important dimensions along which individuals vary. Some of these classification schemes are based on extensive clinical experience, while others are based on statistical methods for identifying clusters.

Wing and Gould (1979) proposed a classification scheme based on the quality of social interactions: aloof, passive, or "active but odd." More recently, Wing (2000) has refined this somewhat by adding a fourth type of social interaction skills, namely those that are learned by higher functioning individuals through verbal rules and memorized strategies, which are then somewhat rigidly and mechanistically applied. In addition to the social interaction variable, she has also identified the variables of verbal skills and nonverbal/practical skills.

A similar approach to classification has been proposed by Tanguay et al. (1998), who suggested that the core deficit in autism is in the social communication domain. Additional variables are presence/absence of mental retardation, and presence/absence of normal language. That is, rather than assuming that difficulties with the formal aspects of language (such as grammar and vocabulary) are a core feature of autism, perhaps they are a related feature, sometimes absent and sometimes present. These authors suggest that this system would eliminate the need for a separate diagnosis of AS: "Autistic persons with normal language are simply autistic persons with normal language" (p. 276).

The analysis by Fein, Rapin, and colleagues (Fein et al., 1999; Rapin, 1996) of a large data set of young children indicated that the basic variable which underlies differences in presentation and developmental course is intelligence (not language delay, as proposed by DSM-IV). Their statistical analysis revealed two distinct groups within the autism spectrum: high functioning and low functioning. They argue that the typical demarcation of these two groups (IQ of 70 or 80) is too high, and suggest that the score to use should be a nonverbal IQ of 65. Even better differentiation could be provided by using three additional factors: the child's Vineland Socialization standard score, score on the Social Abnormalities I scale (provided in both the 1996 and 1999 publications) and age. They indicate that inserting these four variables into a formula provides an overall correct classification rate of 96% (sensitivity of 97% and false positive rate of 5.5%). Almost as accurate, and more clinically practical, is a two-factor formula using nonverbal IQ and Vineland Socialization score, for which they provide a table to determine the probability of the child's membership in the high or low functioning group.

A research group that includes Prior, Eisenmajer, Wing, Gould, and others (1998) has published cluster analysis data supporting a three-cluster division within the autism spectrum. One group seems to correspond to lower-functioning autism, one group to higher-functioning, "Asperger-like" autism, and one group to mild PDD-NOS. They argue that intelligence is not the basis of the differences among the groups, but rather one manifestation of fundamental differences in social and communication impairments. This group explicitly looked at the variables of early language delay and deviance, and found that they did not contribute to the statistical differentiation of the groups, thus undermining the DSM-IV diagnostic criteria.

Eaves et al. (1994) presented a statistical analysis for which they a priori generated four groups. The four groups that emerged were one characterized by severe mental retardation, muteness, and self-abusive behavior; a more typically autistic group with unusual communication and behavior; a higher-functioning, "Asperger-like" group, and another "hard-to-diagnose" group with pragmatic language difficulties, unusual sensory and behavior patterns, and a strong family history of learning problems.

Thus, to date, while there is significant interest in identifying sub-types within the autism spectrum, there is not yet consensus on how many there are or how to define them.

WHAT IS IN A NAME?

If clinically and statistically valid subtypes of autism do exist, what shall we name them? The factor analytic/clustering studies tend to call them Group A, Group B, etc. Clearly this is unsatisfactory outside of a single laboratory or research group. It may well be useful to have a simple name for the subgroup of individuals described as high-functioning/normal language/average IQ/awkwardly sociable. However, as Wing (2000) has pointed out, to use Asperger's name for an empirically-identified group that has significant differences from the children he described is unnecessarily confusing.

Miller and Ozonoff (2000) have described their data as supporting the proposition that AS "may be nothing more than an even milder version of what we already know as high-functioning autism" (p. 236), and question whether a separate name under these circumstances is useful.

In summary, there is not yet professional consensus on how to modify the DSM-IV criteria and terms related to what is currently described as Asperger Syndrome, but undoubtedly changes are coming.

Epilogue

Close to 60 years ago Leo Kanner and Hans Asperger described small samples of the children they were working with from among their much larger pool of patients. Those descriptions were extremely detailed, accurate, and quite provocative. We are not aware of another example in all of child mental health of two papers occurring so close in time to one another, yet unconnected, that have had such an important impact.

Since the papers appeared in print there has been an enormous amount of research, discussion, and speculation about these children. Much of this interest is a tribute to these two fine clinicians because their descriptions were so thoughtful and accurate. A large part of the interest, however, has been because of the children themselves and their remarkable characteristics, strengths, and difficulties. There is something fascinating about the characteristics of people with autism, especially those who are high functioning, that intrigues and captivates us.

In this book we have tried to reflect the fascination but also to offer the solid diagnostic, assessment, and treatment information that has evolved since those seminal papers appeared in the early 1940s. Undoubtedly an incredible amount of information has been collected since that time. Although we now know a lot more about these children (and adults) and how to help them, there is still a long way to go. It is our hope and expectation that books such as this one will help lead to more productive, successful, and meaningful lives for people with AS/HFA, their friends, and their families.

References

Achenbach, T. M. (1991). *The child behavior checklist for ages 4–18*. Burlington, VT: University of Vermont.

Achenbach, T. M., & Rescorla, L. (2000). *The child behavior checklist for ages 1½–5*. Burlington, VT: University of Vermont.

Adams, P. L. (1973). *Obsessive children: A sociopsychiatric study*. London: Brunner/Mazel.

Allen, D. A. (1988). Autistic spectrum disorders: Clinical presentation in preschool children. *Journal of Child Neurology, 3*(Suppl.), 48–56.

Allen, M. H., Lincoln, A. J., & Kaufman, A. S. (1991). Sequential and simultaneous processing abilities of high-functioning autistic and language-impaired children. *Journal of Autism and Developmental Disorders, 21*, 483–502.

American Psychiatric Association. (1980). *Diagnostic and statistical manual of mental disorders* (3rd ed.), Washington, D.C.: Author.

American Psychiatric Association. (1987). *Diagnostic and statistical manual of mental disorders* (3rd ed., rev.), Washington, D.C.: Author.

American Psychiatric Association. (1994). *Diagnostic and statistical manual of mental disorders* (4th ed.), Washington, D.C.: Author.

Asperger, H. (1944/1991). "Autistic Psychopathy" in childhood. In U. Frith (Ed. & Trans.), *Autism and Asperger syndrome* (pp. 37–92). Cambridge: Cambridge University Press. (Original work published 1944).

Asperger, H. (1979). Problems of infantile autism. *Communication, 13*, 45–52.

Attwood, T. (1998). *Asperger's syndrome: A guide for parents and professionals*. Philadelphia: Jessica Kinglsey.

Baltaxe, C. A. M., & Simmons, J. Q. III. (1992). A comparison of language issues in high-functioning autism and related disorders with onset in childhood and adolescence. In E. Schopler & G. B. Mesibov (Eds.), *High functioning individuals with autism* (pp. 201–225). New York: Plenum Press.

Baron-Cohen, S., & Wheelwright, S. (1999). "Obsessions" in children with autism or Asperger's syndrome: Content analysis in terms of core domains of cognition. *British Journal of Psychiatry, 175*, 484–490.

Bartak, L., & Rutter, M. (1976). Differences between mentally retarded and normal intelligence autistic children. *Journal of Autism and Childhood Schizophrenia, 6*, 109–120.

Bennetto, L., Pennington, B. F., & Rogers, S. J. (1995). Intact and impaired memory functions in autism. *Child Development, 67*, 1816–1835.

Berger, H. C., van Spaendonck, P. M., Horstink, M. M., Buytenhuijs, E. L., Lammers, P. M., & Cools, A. R. (1993). Cognitive shifting as a predictor of progress in social understanding in high-functioning adolescents with autism: A prospective study. *Journal of Autism and Developmental Disorders, 23*, 341–359.

Berthier, M. (1995). Hypomania following bereavement in Asperger's syndrome: A case study. *Neuropsychiatry, Neuropsychology, and Behavioral Neurology, 8*, 222–228.

Berument, S. K., Rutter, M., Lord, C., Pickles, A., & Bailey, A. (1999). Autism screening questionnaire: Diagnostic validity. *British Journal of Psychiatry, 175*, 444–451.

Bettelheim, B. (1967). *The empty fortress: Infantile autism and the birth of the self.* London: Collier-Macmillan.

Bishop, D. M. (2000). What's so special about Asperger syndrome? The need for further exploration of the borderlands of autism. In A. Klin, F. R. Volkmar, & S. S. Sparrow (Eds.), *Asperger syndrome* (pp. 254–277). New York: Guilford Press.

Bosch, G. (1970). *Infantile autism.* (D. & I. Jordan, Trans.), New York: Springer-Verlag. (Original work published 1962).

Borys, S. V., Spitz, H. H., & Dorans, B. A. (1982). Tower of Hanoi performance of retarded young adults and nonretarded children as a function of solution length and goal state. *Journal of Experimental Child Psychology, 33*, 87–110.

Boucher, J., & Lewis, V. (1989). Memory impairments and communication in relatively able autistic children. *Journal of Child Psychology and Psychiatry, 30*, 99–122.

Burgoine, E., & Wing, L. (1983). Identical triplets with Asperger's syndrome. *British Journal of Psychiatry, 143*, 261–265.

Carter, A. S., Volkmar, F. R., Sparrow, S. S., Wang, J., Lord, C., Dawson, G., Fombonne, E., Loveland, K., Mesibov, G., & Schopler, E. (1998). The Vineland Adaptive Behavior Scales: Supplementary norms for individuals with autism. *Journal of Autism and Developmental Disabilities, 28*, 287–302.

Church, C., Alisanski, S., & Amanullah, S. (2000). The social, behavioral, and academic experiences of children with Asperger's syndrome. *Focus on Autism and Other Developmental Disabilities, 15*, 12–20.

Dewey, M. (1991). Living with Asperger's syndrome. In U. Frith (Ed.), *Autism and Asperger syndrome* (pp. 184–206). Cambridge: Cambridge University Press.

Dewey, M. A., & Everard, M. P. (1974). The near-normal autistic adolescent. *Journal of Autism and Childhood Schizophrenia, 4*, 348–356.

Dugan, E., Kamps, D., Leonard, B., Watkins, N., Rheinberger, A., & Stackhaus, J. (1995). Effects of cooperative learning groups during social studies for students with autism and fourth-grade peers. *Journal of Applied Behavior Analysis, 28*, 175–188.

Eaves, L. C., Ho, H. H., & Eaves, D. M. (1994). Subtypes of autism by cluster analysis. *Journal of Autism and Developmental Disabilities, 24*, 3–22.

Ehlers, S., Gillberg, C., & Wing, L. (1999). A screening questionnaire for Asperger syndrome and other high-functioning autism spectrum disorders in school age children. *Journal of Autism and Developmental Disabilities, 29*, 129–141.

Ehlers, S., Nyden, A., Gillberg, C., Sandberg, A. D., Dahgren, S., Hjelmquist, E., & Oden, A. (1997). Asperger syndrome, autism, and attention disorders: A comparative study of the cognitive profiles of 120 children. *Journal of Child Psychology and Psychiatry, 38*, 207–217.

Eisenberg, L., & Kanner, L. (1956). Early infantile autism 1943–1955. *American Journal of Orthopsychiatry, 26*, 556–566.

Eisenmajer, R., Prior, M., Leekam, S., Wing, L., Gould, J., Welham, M., & Ong, B. (1996). Comparison of clinical symptoms in autism and Asperger's disorder. *Journal of the American Academy of Child & Adolescent Psychiatry, 35*, 1523–1531.

Eisenmajer, R., Prior, M., Leekam, S., Wing, L., Ong, B., Gould, J., & Welham, M. (1998). Delayed language onset as a predictor of clinical symptoms in pervasive developmental disorders. *Journal of Autism and Developmental Disorders, 28*, 527–533.

Fein, D., Stevens, M., Dunn, M., Waterhouse, L., Allen, D., Rapin, I., & Feinstein, C. (1999). Subtypes of pervasive developmental disorder: Clinical characteristics. *Child Neuropsychology, 5*, 1–23.

Filipek, P. A., Accardo, P. J., Baranek, G. T., Cook, E. H., Dawson, G., Gordon, B., Gravel, J. S., Johnson, C. P., Kallen, R. J., Levy, S. E., Minshew, N. J., Ozonoff, S., Prizant, B. M., Rapin, I., Rogers, S. J., Stone, W. L., Teplin, S., Tuchman, R. F., Volkmar, F. R. (1999). The screening and diagnosis of autistic spectrum disorder. *Journal of Autism and Developmental Disorders, 29*, 439–484.

Freeman, B. J., Lucas, J. C., Forness, S. R., & Ritvo, E. R. (1985). Cognitive processing of high-functioning autistic children: Comparing the K-ABC and WISC-R. *Journal of Psychoeducational Assessment, 4*, 357–362.

Frith, U. (Ed.). (1991). *Autism and Asperger syndrome.* Cambridge: Cambridge University Press.

Fullerton, A., Stratton, J., Coyne, P., & Gray, C. (Eds.) (1996). *Higher functioning adolescents and young adults with autism.* Austin, TX: Pro-ed.

Gagnon, L., Mottron, L., & Joanette, Y. (1997). Questioning the validity of the semantic–pragmatic syndrome diagnosis. *Autism, 1*, 37–55.

Garrison-Harrell, L., Kamps, D., & Kravits, T., (1997). The effects of peer networks on social-communicative behaviors for students with autism. *Focus on Autism and Other Developmental Disabilities, 12*, 241–254.

Ghaziuddin, M., Butler, E., Tsai, L., & Ghaziuddin, N. (1994). Is clumsiness a marker for Asperger syndrome? *Journal of Intellectual Disability Research, 38*, 519–527.

Ghuman, J. K., Freund, L., Reiss, A., Serwint, J., & Folstein, S. (1998). Early detection of social interaction problems: Development of a social interaction instrument in young children. *Journal of Developmental and Behavioral Pediatrics, 19*, 411–419.

Gillberg, C. (1989). Asperger syndrome in 23 Swedish children. *Developmental Medicine and Child Neurology, 31*, 520–531.

Goldstein, G., Minshew, N. J., & Siegel, D. J. (1994). Age differences in academic achievement in high-functioning autistic individuals. *Journal of Clinical and Experimental Neuropsychology, 16*, 671–680.

Grandin, T. (1995). *Thinking in pictures and other reports from my life with autism.* New York: Doubleday.

Gray, C. (1998). Social stories and comic strip conversations with students with Asperger syndrome and high-functioning autism. In E. Schopler, G. B. Mesibov, & L. J. Kunce (Eds.), *Asperger syndrome or high-functioning autism?* (pp. 167–198). New York: Plenum Press.

Hare, D. G. (1997). The use of cognitive behavioural therapy with people with Asperger syndrome. *Autism, 1,* 215–225.

Harris, S., Handleman, J., & Burton, J. (1990). The Stanford Binet profiles of young children with autism. *Special Services in the School, 6,* 135–143.

Kamps, D. M., Barbetta, P. M., Leonard, B. R., & Delquadri, J. (1994). Classwide peer tutoring: An integration strategy to improve reading skills and promote peer interactions among students with autism and general education peers. *Journal of Applied Behavior Analysis, 27,* 49–61.

Kamps, D. M., Leonard, B., Potucek, J., & Garrison-Harrell, L. (1995). Cooperative learning groups in reading: An integration strategy for students with autism and general classroom peers. *Behavioral Disorders, 21,* 89–109.

Kanner, L. (1943). Autistic disturbances of affective content. *Nervous Child, 2,* 217–250.

Kinsbourne, M., & Caplan, P. J. (1979). *Children's learning and attention problems.* Boston: Little, Brown & Co.

Kirkman, M., Kirk, U., & Kemp, S. (1998). *NEPSY: A developmental neuropsychological assessment.* San Antonio, TX: The Psychological Corporation.

Klin, A., Sparrow, S. S., Marans, W. D., Carter, A., & Volkmar, F. R. (2000). Assessment issues in children and adolescents with Asperger syndrome. In A. Klin, F. R. Volkmar, & S. S. Sparrow (Eds.), *Asperger syndrome* (pp. 309–339). New York: Guilford Press.

Klin, A., Sparrow, S. S., Volkmar, F. R., Cicchetti, D. V., & Rourke, B. P. (1995). Asperger syndrome. In B. P. Rourke (Ed.), *Syndrome of nonverbal learning disabilities: Neurodevelopmental manifestations* (pp. 93–118). New York: Guilford Press.

Klin, A., Volkmar, F. R., & Sparrow, S. S. (2000). Introduction. In A. Klin, F. R. Volkmar, & S. S. Sparrow (Eds.), *Asperger syndrome* (pp. 1–21). New York: Guilford Press.

Klin, A., Volkmar, F. R., Sparrow, S. S., Cicchetti, D. V., & Rourke, B. P. (1995). Validity and neuropsychological characterization of Asperger syndrome: Convergence with nonverbal learning disabilities syndrome. *Journal of Child Psychology and Psychiatry, 38,* 1127–1140.

Koegel, R. L. & Frea, W. D. (1993). Treatment of social behavior in autism through the modification of pivotal social skills. *Journal of Applied Behavior Analysis, 26,* 369–377.

Kretschmer, E. (1925). *Physique and character.* New York: Harcourt, Brace & Co.

Kunce, L., & Mesibov, G. B. (1998). Educational approaches to high-functioning autism and Asperger Syndrome. In E. Schopler, G. B. Mesibov, & L. Kunce (Eds.), *Asperger syndrome or high-functioning autism?* (pp. 227–261). New York: Plenum.

Landa, R. (2000). Social language use in Asperger syndrome and high-functioning autism. In A. Klin, F. R. Volkmar, & S. S. Sparrow (Eds.), *Asperger syndrome* (pp. 159–171). New York: Guilford Press.

Lincoln, A. J., Allen, M. H., & Kilman, A. (1995). The assessment and interpretation of intellectual abilities in people with autism. In E. Schopler, & G. B. Mesibov (Eds.), *Learning and cognition in autism* (pp. 89–117). New York: Plenum Press.

Lincoln, A. J., Courchenese, E., Allen, M., Hanson, E., & Ene, M. (1998). Neuro-biology of Asperger syndrome: Seven case studies and quantitative magnetic resonance imaging findings. In E. Schopler, G. B. Mesibov, & L. J. Kunce (Eds.), *Asperger syndrome or high-functioning autism?* (pp. 145–163). New York: Plenum Press.

Lord, C., Risi, S., Lambrecht, L., Cook, E. H., Jr., Leventhal, B. D., DiLavore, P. C., Pickles, A., & Rutter, M. (2000). The autism diagnostic observation scale–generic: A standard measure of social and communication deficits associated with the spectrum of autism. *Journal of Autism and Developmental Disorders, 30*, 205–223.

Lord, C., Rutter, M., & Le Couteur, A. (1994). Autism diagnostic interview-revised: A revised version of a diagnostic interview for caregivers of individuals with possible pervasive developmetal disorders. *Journal of Autism and Developmental Disorders, 24*, 659–685.

Lord, C., & Venter, A. (1992). Outcome and follow-up studies of high-functioning autistic individuals. In E. Schopler, & G. B. Mesibov (Eds.), *High-functioning individuals with autism* (pp. 187–199). New York: Plenum Press.

Manjiviona, J., & Prior, M. (1995). Comparison of Asperger syndrome and high-functioning autistic children on a test of motor impairment. *Journal of Autism and Developmental Disorders, 25*, 23–39.

Manjiviona, J., & Prior, M. (1999). Neuropsychological profiles of children with Asperger syndrome and autism. *Autism, 3*, 327–356.

Marans, W. D. (1997). Developmentally Based Assessments [Section 19.3.]. In D. J. Cohen, & F. R. Volkmar (Eds.), *Handbook of autism and pervasive developmental disorders* (2nd edition., pp. 427–441). New York: John Wiley & Sons.

Marriage, K. J., Gordon, V., & Brand, L. (1995). A social skills group for boys with Asperger's syndrome. *Australian and New Zealand Journal of Psychiatry, 29*, 58–62.

McDougle, C. J., Kresch, L. E., Goodman, W. K., & Naylor, S. T. (1995). A case-controlled study of repetitive thoughts and behavior in adults with autistic disorder and obsessive-compulsive disorder. *American Journal of Psychiatry, 152*, 772–777.

Mesibov, G. B. (1994). A comprehensive program for serving people with autism and their families: The TEACCH model. In J. L. Matson (Eds.), *Autism in children and adults: Etiology, assessment, and intervention* (pp. 85–97). Belmont, CA: Brooks/Cole.

Mesibov, G. B., Adams, L. W., & Klinger, L. G. (1998). *Autism: Understanding the disorder*. New York: Plenum.

Mesibov, G. B., Schopler, E., & Hearsey, K. A. (1994). Structured teaching. In E. Schopler & G. B. Mesibov (Eds.), *Behavioral issues in autism* (pp. 193–205). New York: Plenum.

Miller, J. N., & Ozonoff, S. (1997). Did Asperger's cases have Asperger disorder? A research note. *Journal of Child Psychology and Psychiatry, 38,* 247–251.

Miller, J. N., & Ozonoff, S. (2000). The external validity of Asperger disorder: Lack of evidence from the domain of neuropsychology. *Journal of Abnormal Psychology, 109,* 227–238.

Minshew, N. M., Goldstein, G., Muenz, L. R., & Payton, J. (1992). Neuropsychological functioning in nonmentally retarded autistic individuals. *Journal of Clinical and Experimental Neuropsychology, 14,* 749–761.

Minshew, N. M., Goldstein, G., & Siegel, D. J. (1995). Speech and language in high-functioning autistic individuals. *Neuropsychology, 9,* 255–261.

Minshew, N. J., Goldstein, G., & Siegel, D. J. (1997). Neuropsychologic functioning in autism: Profile of a complex information processing disorder. *Journal of the International Neuropsychological Society, 3,* 303–316.

Minshew, N. J., Goldstein, G., Taylor, G. H., & Siegel, D. J. (1994). Academic achievement in high functioning autistic individuals. *Journal of Clinical and Experimental Neuropsychology, 16,* 261–270.

Moreno, S. J. (1991) High-functioning individuals with autism: Advice and information for parents and others who care. Crown Point, IN: MAAP Services (PO Box 524, Crown Point, IN 46307).

Myles, B. S., & Simpson, R. L. (1998). *Asperger syndrome: A guide for educators and parents.* Austin, TX: Pro-Ed.

Naglieri, J. A., Kamphaus, R. W., & Kaufman, A. S. (1983). The Luria-Das successive-simultaneous model applied to the WISC-R data. *Journal of Psychoeducational Assessment, 1,* 25–34.

Ozonoff, S. (1995). Reliability and validity studies of the Wisconsin Card Sorting Test studies of autism. *Neuropsychology, 9,* 491–500.

Ozonoff, S. (1998). Assessment and remediation of executive dysfunction in autism and Asperger syndrome. In E. Schopler, G. B. Mesibov, & L. J. Kunce (Eds.), *Asperger syndrome or high-functioning autism?* (pp. 263–289). New York: Plenum Press.

Ozonoff, S., & Griffith, E. M. (2000). Neuropsychological function and the external validity of Asperger syndrome. In A. Klin, F. R. Volkmar, & S. S. Sparrow (Eds.), *Asperger syndrome* (pp. 72–96). New York: Guilford Press.

Ozonoff, S., & Jensen, J. (1999). Brief report: Specific executive function profiles in three neurodevelopmental disorders. *Journal of Autism and Developmental Disorders, 29,* 171–177.

Ozonoff, S., Pennington, B. F., & Rogers, S. J. (1991). Executive function deficits in high-functioning autistic individuals: Relationship to theory of mind. *Journal of Child Psychology and Psychiatry and Allied Disciplines, 32,* 1081–1105.

Ozonoff, S., Rogers, S. J., & Pennington, B. F. (1991). Asperger's syndrome: Evidence of an empirical distinction from high-functioning autism. *Journal of Child Psychology and Psychiatry, 32,* 1107–1122.

Ozonoff, S., South, M., & Miller, J. N. (2000). DSM-IV-defined Asperger syndrome: Cognitive, behavioral and early history differentiation from high-functioning autism. *Autism, 4*, 29–46.

Prior, M., Eisenmajer, R., Leekam, S., Wing, L., Gould, J., Ong, B., & Dowe, D. (1998). Are there subgroups within the autistic spectrum? A cluster analysis of a group of children with autistic spectrum disorders. *Journal of Child Psychology and Psychiatry, 39*, 893–902.

Prizant, B. M. & Rydell, P. J. (1984). Analysis of functions of delayed echolalia in autistic children. *Journal of Speech & Hearing Research, 27*, 183–192.

Rapin, I. (editor for the Autism and Language Disorders Collaborative Project: Preschool Study Group) (1996). Preschool children with inadequate communication: Developmental language disorder, autism, low IQ. *Clinics in Developmental Medicine, 139*, London: Mac Keith Press.

Robinson, J. F., & Vitale, L. J. (1954). Children with circumscribed interest patterns. *American Journal of Orthopsychiatry, 24*, 755–766.

Rosenblatt, J., Bloom, P., & Koegel, R. L. (1995). Overselective responding: Description, implications, and intervention. In R. L. Koegel & L. K. Koegel (Eds.). *Teaching children with autism: Strategies for initiating positive interactions and improving learning opportunities.* (pp. 33–42). Baltimore: P.H. Brookes Publishing Co.

Rourke, B. P. (1989). *Nonverbal learning disabilities: The syndrome and the model.* New York: Guilford Press.

Rourke, B. P. (1995). Introduction: The NLD syndrome and the white matter model. In B. P. Rourke (Ed.), *Syndrome of nonverbal learning disabilities: Neurodevelopmental manifestations.* (pp. 1–26). New York: Guilford Press.

Rourke, B. P., & Tsatsanis, K. D. (2000). Nonverbal learning disabilities and Asperger syndrome. In A. Klin, F. R. Volkmar, & S. S. Sparrow (Eds.), *Asperger syndrome* (pp. 231–253). New York: Guilford Press.

Rumsey, J. M. (1985). Conceptual problem-solving in highly verbal, nonretarded autistic men. *Journal of Autism and Developmental Disorders, 15*, 23–36.

Rumsey, J. M., & Hamburger, S. D. (1988). Neuropsychological findings in high-functioning men with infantile autism, residual state. *Journal of Clinical and Experimental Neuropsychology, 10*, 201–221.

Rumsey, J. M., & Hamburger, S. D. (1990). Neuropsychological divergence of high-level autism and severe dyslexia. *Journal of Autism and Developmental Disorders, 20*, 155–168.

Rutter, M., & Bartak, L. (1973). Special education treatment of autistic children: A comparative study–II. Follow-up findings and implications for services. *Journal of Child Psychology and Psychiatry, 14*, 241–270.

Rutter, M., & Schopler, E. (Eds.) (1978). *Autism: A reappraisal of concepts and treatment.* New York: Plenum.

Schopler, E. (1994). Behavioral priorities for autism and related developmental disorders. In E. Schopler & G. B. Mesibov (Eds.). *Behavioral issues in autism.* New York: Plenum Press.

Shea, V. (1984). Explaining mental retardation and autism to parents. In E. Schopler & G. B. Mesibov (Eds.), *The effects of autism on the family.* (pp. 265–288). New York: Plenum Press.

Shea, V. (1993). Interpreting results to parents of preschool children. In E. Schopler, M. E. Van Bourgondien, & M. Bristol (Eds.), *Preschool issues in autism* (pp. 195–203). New York: Plenum Press.

Shea, V., & Mesibov, G. B. (1985). Brief Report: The relationship of learning disabilities and higher-level autism. *Journal of Autism and Developmental Disorders, 15*, 425–435.

Siegel, D. J., Minshew, N. M., & Goldstein, G. (1996). Wechsler IQ profiles in diagnosis of high-functioning autism. *Journal of Autism and Developmental Disorders, 26*, 389–406.

Swaggart, B. L., Gagnon, E., Bock, S. J., Earles, T. L., Quinn, C. Myles, B. S., & Simpson, R. L. (1995) Using social stories to teach social and behavioral skills to children with autism. *Focus on Autistic Behavior, 1*, 1–16.

Szatmari, P. (1998). Differential diagnosis of Asperger disorder. In E. Schopler, G. B. Mesibov, & L. J. Kunce (Eds.), *Asperger syndrome or high-functioning autism?* (pp. 61–76). New York: Plenum Press.

Szatmari, P. (2000). Perspectives on the classification of Asperger syndrome. In A. Klin, F. R. Volkmar, & S. S. Sparrow (Eds.), *Asperger syndrome* (pp. 403–417). New York: Guilford Press.

Szatmari, P., Archer, L., Fisman, S., Steiner, D. L., & Wilson, F. (1995). Asperger's syndrome and autism: Differences in behavior, cognition, and adaptive functioning. *Journal of the American Academy of Child and Adolescent Psychiatry, 34*, 1662–1671.

Szatmari, P., Tuff, L., Finlayson, A. J., & Bartolucci, G. (1989). Asperger syndrome and autism: Neurocognitive aspects. *Journal of American Academy of Child and Adolescent Psychiatry, 29*, 130–136.

Tanguay, P. E., Robertson, J., & Derrick, A. (1998). A dimensional classification of autism spectrum disorder by social communication domains. *Journal of the American Academy of Child & Adolescent Psychiatry, 37*, 271–277.

Twachtman-Cullen, D. (1998). Language and communication in high functioning autism and Asperger syndrome. In E. Schopler, G. B. Mesibov, & L. J. Kunce (Eds.), *Asperger syndrome or high-functioning autism?* (pp. 199–225). New York: Plenum Press.

Van Krevelen, D. A. (1971). Early infantile autism and autistic psychopathology. *Journal of Autism and Childhood Schizophrenia, 1*(1), 82–86.

Van Krevelen, D. A., & Kuipers, C. (1962). The psychopathology of autistic psychopathy. *Acta Paedopsychiatrica, 29*, 22–31.

Volkmar, F. R. (1997). Ask the editor. *Journal of Autism and Developmental Disorders, 27*, 103–105.

Volkmar, F. R., & Klin, A. (1998). Asperger syndrome and nonverbal learning disabilities. In E. Schopler, G. B. Mesibov, & L. J. Kunce (Eds.), *Asperger syndrome or high-functioning autism?* (pp. 107–121). New York: Plenum Press.

Volkmar, F. R., & Klin, A. (2000). Diagnostic issues in Asperger syndrome. In A. Klin, F. R. Volkmar, & S. S. Sparrow (Eds.), *Asperger syndrome* (pp. 25–71). New York: Guilford Press.

Williams, D. (1998). *Autism: An inside-out approach.* London: Jessica Kingsley.

Williams, K. (1995). Understanding the student with Asperger syndrome: Guidelines for teachers. [On-line]. Available: http://www.udel.edu/bkirby/asperger

Williams, T. I. (1989). A social skills group for autistic children. *Journal of Autism and Developmental Disorders, 19,* 143–155.

Wing, L. (1976). Diagnosis, clinical description, and prognosis. In L. Wing (Ed.). *Early childhood autism: Clinical, educational, and social aspects* (2nd ed., pp. 15–64). Oxford: Pergamon.

Wing, L. (1981). Asperger's syndrome: A clinical account. *Psychological Medicine, 11,* 115–129.

Wing, L. (1986). Clarification on Asperger's Syndrome [Letter to the Editor]. *Journal of Autism and Developmental Disorders, 16,* 513–515.

Wing, L., (1988). The continuum of autistic characteristics. In E. Schopler & G. B. Mesibov (Eds.), *Diagnosis and assessment in autism.* (pp. 91–110). New York: Plenum.

Wing, L. (1998). The history of Asperger syndrome. In E. Schopler, G. B. Mesibov, & L. J. Kunce (Eds.), *Asperger syndrome or high-functioning autism?* (pp. 12–28). New York: Plenum Press.

Wing, L. (2000). Past and future of research on Asperger syndrome. In A. Klin, F. R. Volkmar, & S. S. Sparrow (Eds.), *Asperger syndrome* (pp. 418–432). New York: Guilford Press.

Wing, L., & Gould, J. (1979). Severe impairments of social interaction and associated abnormalities in children: Epidemiology and classification. *Journal of Autism and Developmental Disorders, 9,* 11–29.

Wolff, S. (1998). Schizoid personality in childhood: The links with Asperger syndrome, schizophrenia spectrum disorders, and elective mutism. In E. Schopler, G. B. Mesibov, & L. J. Kunce (Eds.), *Asperger syndrome or high-functioning autism?* (pp. 123–142). New York: Prenum Press.

Wolff, S. (2000). Schizoid personality in childhood and Asperger syndrome. In A. Klin, F. R. Volkmar, & S. S. Sparrow (Eds.), *Asperger syndrome* (pp. 278–305). New York: Guilford Press.

Wolff, S. & Barlow, A. (1979). Schizoid personality in childhood: A comparative study of schizoid, autistic, and normal children. *Journal of Child Psychology and Psychiatry, 20,* 29–46.

Wolff, S. & Chick, J. (1980). Schizoid personality in childhood: A controlled follow-up study. *Psychological Medicine, 10,* 85–100.

World Health Organization. (1992). *The ICD-10 classification of mental and behavioural disorders: Clinical descriptions and diagnostic guidelines.* Geneva: WHO.

Yirmiya, N., & Sigman, M. (1991). High functioning individuals with autism: Diagnosis, empirical findings, and theoretical issues. *Clinical Psychology Review, 11,* 669–683.

Index